Type 2 Diabetes Cookbook
Beginner's Quick & Easy Recipes for Delicious Diabetes Diets

AF885288

300 Healthy

<u>Dinners</u>

for

Diabetic Wellness in 30 minutes or Less

By

Lily Anders

Copyright Page

Ace East Publishing LLC
1401 21st Street
Suite R
Sacramento, CA 95811

ISBN: **978-1-963939-82-8**

First Edition

ACE EAST
PUBLISHING

Disclaimer Page

This cookbook is crafted to offer insightful information and recipes for those interested in managing Type 2 Diabetes through dietary choices. It is important to recognize that the authors and the publisher are not healthcare professionals. The suggestions and recipes contained within this book are not meant to replace professional medical advice, diagnoses, or treatments. Should you have any healthcare-related questions or concerns, particularly relating to Type 2 Diabetes management, we strongly advise consulting with your doctor or a qualified healthcare provider.

The culinary experiences, and recommendations shared in this book stem from extensive research and the personal journey of exploring dietary approaches to Type 2 Diabetes management. These narratives and suggestions are intended for educational and motivational purposes only, aiming to enhance understanding and inspire positive lifestyle changes, not to serve as direct medical or nutritional prescriptions.

The author(s) and publisher expressly disclaim any liability for any adverse effects arising directly or indirectly from the use and application of the information contained in this cookbook. Moreover, given the specificity and medical relevance of the content, certain topics and dietary advice may not be suitable for all readers. It is advisable for caregivers and adults to review the content before sharing with minors or individuals with particular sensitivities or health concerns.

In cases of medical emergencies or for immediate assistance with health issues, please reach out to a trusted healthcare professional or dial the emergency services number available in your locality.

The Entire Type 2 Diabetes Cookbook Series

Dive into a culinary revolution with the ***"Type 2 Diabetes Cookbook Series: Beginner's Quick & Easy Recipes for Delicious Diabetes Diets – 300 Health-Boosting Savory Meals for Diabetic Wellness in 30 Minutes or Less."***

Spread across six essential volumes – Breakfast, Lunch, Dinner, Desserts, Snacks, and Sauces, Dips, & Dressings – this series is your passport to a world where managing Type 2 Diabetes meets delicious innovation.

Each book is a treasure trove of hundreds of recipes, marrying the precision of nutritional science with the flair of culinary art. Designed for those on a diabetic diet, these recipes promise to transform your meals from bland to blissful without sacrificing flavor or health. Every dish, from energizing breakfasts to indulgent desserts, comes alive through vivid, full-color photographs, accompanied by foolproof instructions, cooking times, detailed ingredient lists, serving suggestions, and handy conversion charts.

But the journey doesn't end with tantalizing meals. These cookbooks are gateways to mastering diabetes management, offering insights into blood sugar balance, insulin functionality, and the art of carb counting. They stand as pillars of empowerment and knowledge, guiding you through the culinary and health aspects of diabetes with ease and enjoyment.

Embrace these cookbooks as more than mere collections of recipes; see them as companions in your journey toward diabetic wellness, bringing confidence, pleasure, and a burst of flavors into your daily life. Step into a world where managing diabetes is synonymous with culinary discovery and dietary joy. Welcome to your new kitchen adventure!

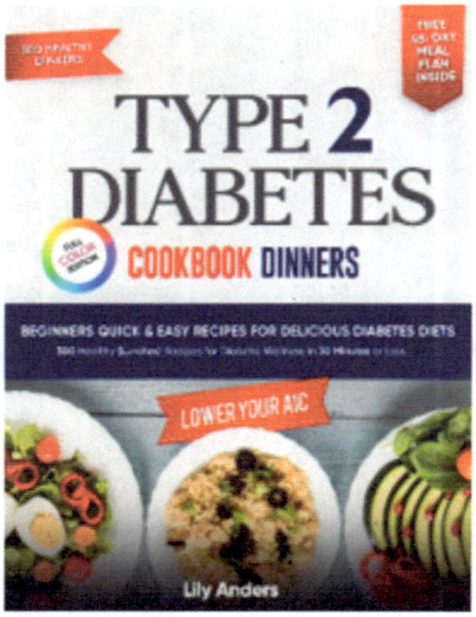
TYPE 2
DIABETES
COOKBOOK DINNERS
BEGINNERS QUICK & EASY RECIPES FOR DELICIOUS DIABETES DIETS
LOWER YOUR A1C
Lily Anders

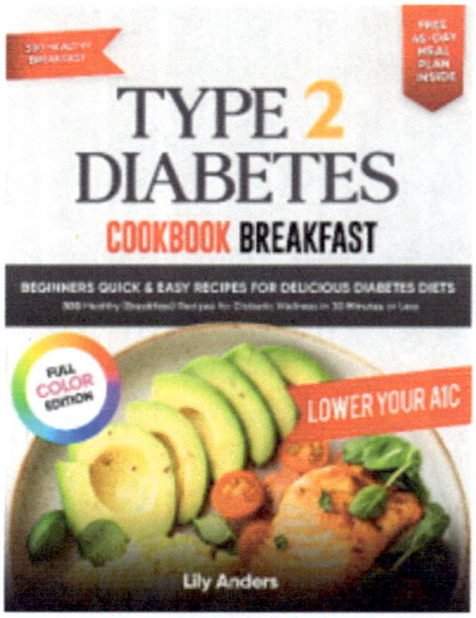
TYPE 2
DIABETES
COOKBOOK BREAKFAST
BEGINNERS QUICK & EASY RECIPES FOR DELICIOUS DIABETES DIETS
FULL COLOR EDITION
LOWER YOUR A1C
Lily Anders

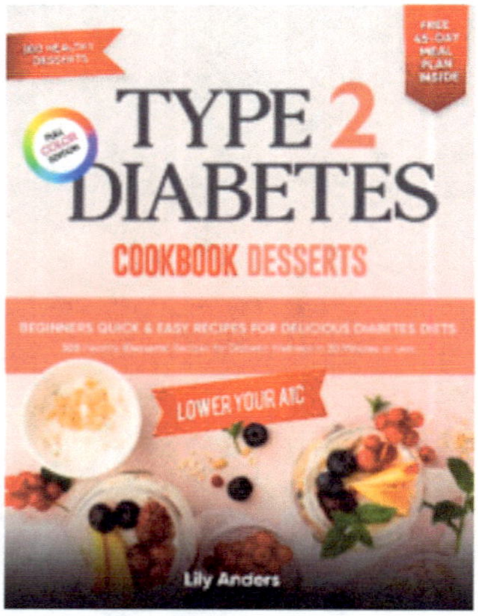
TYPE 2
DIABETES
COOKBOOK DESSERTS
BEGINNERS QUICK & EASY RECIPES FOR DELICIOUS DIABETES DIETS
LOWER YOUR A1C
Lily Anders

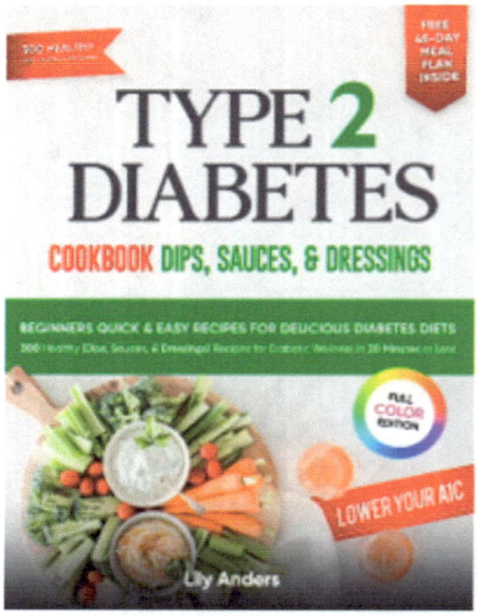
TYPE 2
DIABETES
COOKBOOK DIPS, SAUCES, & DRESSINGS
BEGINNERS QUICK & EASY RECIPES FOR DELICIOUS DIABETES DIETS
FULL COLOR EDITION
LOWER YOUR A1C
Lily Anders

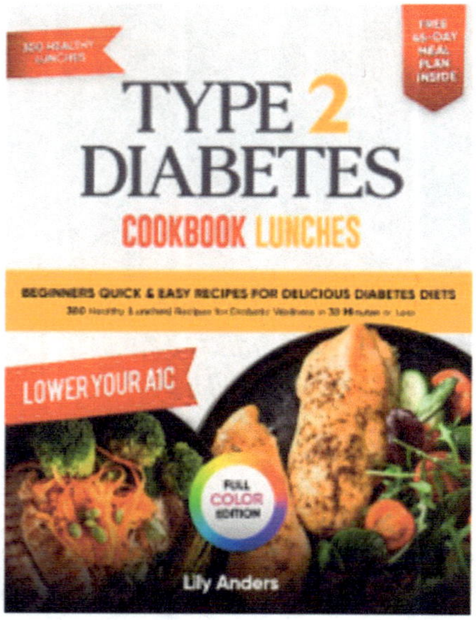
TYPE 2
DIABETES
COOKBOOK LUNCHES
BEGINNERS QUICK & EASY RECIPES FOR DELICIOUS DIABETES DIETS
LOWER YOUR A1C
FULL COLOR EDITION
Lily Anders

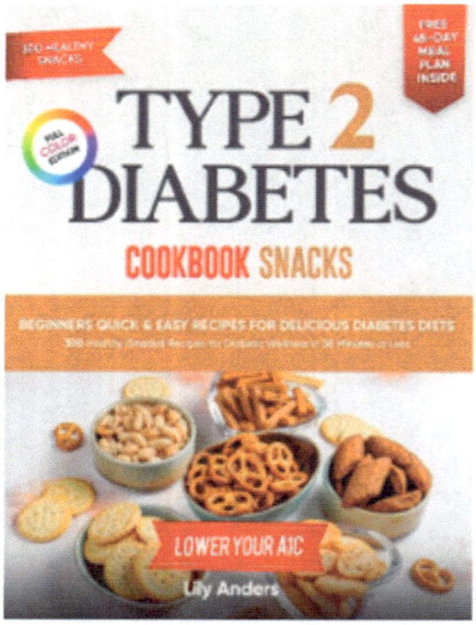
TYPE 2
DIABETES
COOKBOOK SNACKS
BEGINNERS QUICK & EASY RECIPES FOR DELICIOUS DIABETES DIETS
LOWER YOUR A1C
Lily Anders

Here's My Promise to You!

To jumpstart your journey toward healthier eating, here are the remaining

Listing of 200 Delicious & Diabetes-Friendly Dinner Recipes!

That's right—you now have access to a treasure trove of 200 additional diabetic recipes designed to help you enjoy flavorful, balanced meals while managing your blood sugar with confidence. These Dinner recipes will inspire you to create satisfying, nutritious meals with ease.

☞ CLICK THE LINK OR SCAN THE QR CODE TO DOWNLOAD YOUR FREE RECIPE COLLECTION!

Enjoy, and Happy Cooking!

The journey to better health starts with the right food choices, and this cookbook and it is here to support you every step of the way.

Thank you for trusting this guide, and here's to a flavorful, balanced, and empowered approach to managing Type 2 Diabetes!

You've got this! □□✨

<<Click here to access your 45-day meal plan>>

https://acrobat.adobe.com/id/urn:aaid:sc:VA6C2:448a7fa7-ffcd-4919-9d29-1c8e6bee62e9

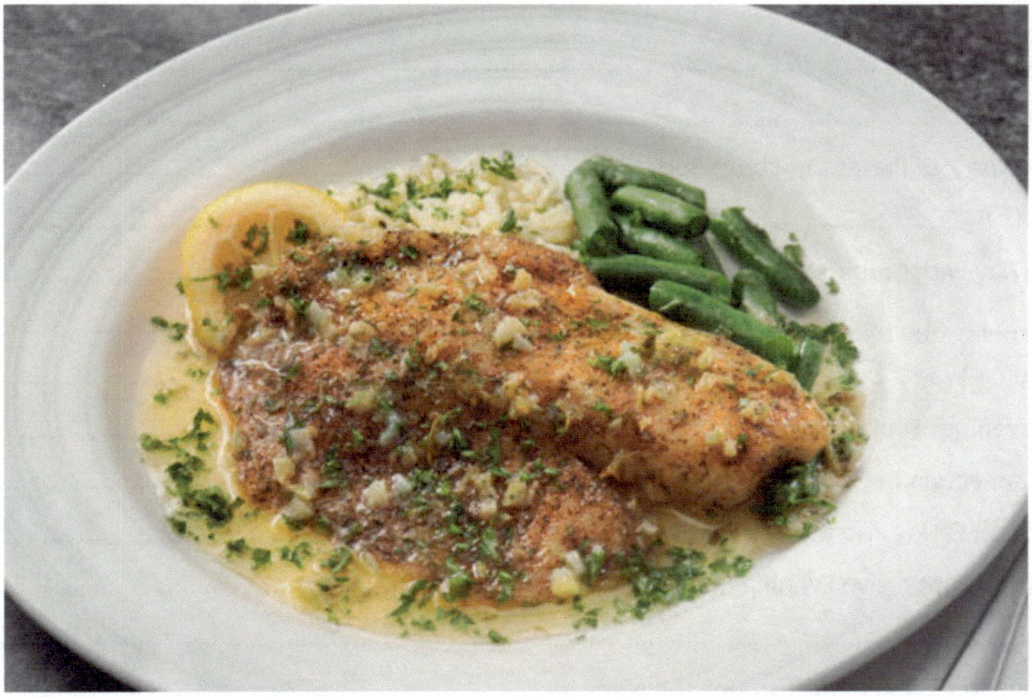

1. Lemon Garlic Grilled Tilapia with Roasted Asparagus

Prep.Time: 15 min	Cook Time: 10-12 min	Serving: 2	Beverage pairing: Iced Tea

Ingredients:

- 2 tilapia fillets
- 2 cloves garlic, minced
- 1 lemon, juiced and zested
- 1 tablespoon olive oil
- Salt and pepper to taste
- 1 bunch asparagus, trimmed
- Cooking spray

Preparation:

1. Preheat the grill to medium-high heat.
2. In a small bowl, mix minced garlic, lemon juice, lemon zest, olive oil, salt, and pepper.
3. Place tilapia fillets in a shallow dish and pour the lemon garlic marinade over them. Allow them to marinate for 15-20 minutes.
4. Meanwhile, preheat the oven to 400°F (200°C). Place the trimmed asparagus on a baking sheet, spray with cooking spray, and sprinkle with salt and pepper. Roast in the oven for 10-12 minutes, or until tender.
5. Grill the marinated tilapia fillets for 3-4 minutes per side, or until cooked through and flaky.
6. Serve the grilled tilapia alongside the roasted asparagus.

Nutrition Facts (per serving):

- Calories: 250
- Carbs: 9g
- Protein: 35g
- Fat: 8g

Table of Contents

INTRODUCTION

Ending the Day with Confidence and Balance

By the time dinner arrives, many people managing Type 2 Diabetes feel worn down. The day has been long, energy is low, and hunger is strong. Decisions that felt manageable earlier now feel heavier, and food choices can feel rushed or overwhelming.

Dinner often becomes the most emotionally loaded meal of the day.

It is where fatigue meets appetite, and where the pressure to make the "right" choice can feel strongest. Convenience foods, oversized portions, and carbohydrate-heavy meals may seem comforting in the moment, but they often lead to blood sugar spikes, discomfort, or regret later in the evening.

This book was written for that moment.

The Type 2 Diabetes Cookbook: Dinner is designed to bring calm and clarity back to your evenings. It focuses on balanced, satisfying meals that support blood sugar stability while still feeling like real dinners you can enjoy at the end of a long day.

Dinner plays a unique role in managing Type 2 Diabetes. It influences overnight blood sugar levels, sleep quality, and how you feel the next morning. A well-balanced evening meal can help the body wind down, reduce late-night cravings, and support more stable mornings ahead.

The good news is that diabetes-friendly dinners do not need to be bland, restrictive, or time-consuming.

Inside this book, you will find practical dinner recipes created to be comforting without excess and nourishing without complexity. Meals are designed to be prepared in 30 minutes or less and built around thoughtful combinations of protein, vegetables, and controlled carbohydrates.

This cookbook is not about rigid rules or perfect execution. It is about creating evening meals that feel grounding and dependable. Whether you are cooking for yourself or sharing dinner with others, these recipes are meant to fit into real life.

You will not be asked to give up flavor or enjoyment. Instead, you will learn how to structure dinners that leave you feeling satisfied rather than overly full, supported rather than restricted.

Most importantly, this book is meant to help you end each day with confidence instead of uncertainty.

Dinner should be a moment to pause, nourish your body, and prepare for rest.

Welcome to a calmer, more balanced way to close your day.

Chapter 1

Understanding Type 2 Diabetes in the Evening

As the day winds down, the body begins to shift into a different rhythm. Energy demands change, activity levels often decrease, and digestion slows. For individuals managing Type 2 Diabetes, these evening changes can influence how food is processed and how blood sugar behaves overnight.

Type 2 Diabetes affects the body's ability to use insulin efficiently. Insulin helps move glucose from the bloodstream into the cells, where it can be used for energy. When insulin does not function as effectively as it should, glucose remains in the blood longer, leading to elevated blood sugar levels.

In the evening, this process can become more noticeable.

Why Evenings Feel Different

By dinner time, the body has already responded to the foods, movement, and stress of the day. Blood sugar levels may have fluctuated, insulin has been active for many hours, and fatigue can influence appetite and food choices.

As activity levels decrease in the evening, the body may become less efficient at processing large or unbalanced meals. This makes dinner an important opportunity to support blood sugar stability rather than disrupt it.

Large portions, heavy carbohydrates, or meals eaten late at night can cause blood sugar levels to remain elevated longer than intended. This may affect sleep quality and contribute to higher morning blood sugar readings.

The Connection Between Dinner and Overnight Blood Sugar

Dinner not only affects the evening hours. It plays a role in what happens overnight and how the body feels the next morning.

Balanced dinners that include protein, fiber, and moderate carbohydrates help promote steadier blood sugar levels during sleep. When digestion is slower and more controlled, the body can rest more effectively.

In contrast, meals that are overly large or carbohydrate-heavy may lead to discomfort, late-night hunger, or restless sleep. These patterns can make blood sugar management feel more difficult the following day.

Emotional Eating and the End of the Day

Evenings often carry emotional weight. Stress, fatigue, and the desire for comfort can influence how and what we eat. This is especially common at dinner, when food is often used as a way to relax or reward oneself after a long day.

Understanding this emotional context is important. Managing Type 2 Diabetes does not mean ignoring these feelings. It means acknowledging them and creating dinner routines that feel supportive rather than restrictive.

This book focuses on dinners that provide comfort through balance, flavor, and satisfaction, without excess.

Building a Supportive Evening Routine

Consistency at dinner helps reinforce overall blood sugar management. When evening meals are predictable and balanced, the body responds with improved regulation.

This does not require rigid schedules or identical meals each night. It requires thoughtful structure and an understanding of how the evening environment affects food choices.

By approaching dinner with intention, you create a foundation for better rest, steadier mornings, and greater confidence in managing Type 2 Diabetes.

In the next chapter, we will explore how blood sugar behaves after dinner and why certain evening meals help prevent nighttime spikes and next-day challenges.

Chapter 2

Blood Sugar After Dinner and Through the Night

Dinner marks the final major meal of the day, and its effects often extend well beyond the evening hours. For individuals managing Type 2 Diabetes, what happens after dinner plays an important role in overnight blood sugar patterns, sleep quality, and how the body feels the next morning.

After eating dinner, blood sugar levels rise as food is digested and glucose enters the bloodstream. Insulin is released to help move this glucose into the cells. When dinner is balanced, this process occurs gradually. When dinner is heavy or unbalanced, blood sugar levels may remain elevated longer than intended.

How Evening Meals Affect Overnight Blood Sugar

In the evening, physical activity tends to decrease. With less movement to help use glucose, the body may take longer to process carbohydrates consumed at dinner. This makes the composition and portion size of evening meals especially important.

Meals that are high in refined carbohydrates or large in portion size can lead to prolonged blood sugar elevations. These elevations may continue into the night, affecting sleep and contributing to higher fasting blood sugar levels in the morning.

Balanced dinners that include protein, fiber, and controlled carbohydrates support a more stable blood sugar response. When digestion is slower and more predictable, the body can settle into rest more effectively.

The Relationship Between Dinner and Sleep

Blood sugar levels influence sleep quality more than many people realize. Fluctuations in blood sugar during the night may cause restlessness, frequent waking, or discomfort.

Eating very late, overeating, or choosing heavy meals can interfere with the body's natural ability to wind down. This may lead to disrupted sleep and fatigue the next day.

Dinners that are satisfying without being heavy help support better sleep by allowing the body to digest efficiently before rest.

Late-Night Hunger and Evening Snacking

Late-night hunger is common, especially when dinner lacks balance. Meals that are low in protein or fiber may leave you feeling hungry shortly after eating.

This can lead to unplanned evening snacking, which may further impact blood sugar levels overnight. Addressing dinner balance helps reduce the likelihood of late-night cravings.

When hunger does arise, it is often a sign that dinner composition or timing needs adjustment rather than restriction.

Creating a Calmer Evening Pattern

Dinner sets the tone for the final hours of the day. Balanced meals help signal to the body that nourishment has been provided, allowing systems to slow down naturally.

Establishing consistent dinner habits supports better blood sugar regulation and promotes a smoother transition into sleep.

This book emphasizes dinners that help you feel settled rather than stimulated. Meals are designed to nourish without overloading the body late in the day.

In the next chapter, we will focus on carbohydrates at dinner, how to approach them thoughtfully, and how to include them without disrupting overnight balance.

Chapter 3

Carbohydrates at Dinner Without Disruption

Carbohydrates at dinner often create uncertainty for individuals managing Type 2 Diabetes. After a long day, carbohydrate-rich foods can feel comforting and familiar, yet they are frequently associated with nighttime blood sugar concerns. This tension can lead to either avoidance or overconsumption, neither of which supports balance.

The goal at dinner is not to eliminate carbohydrates. It is to include them thoughtfully, in portions and combinations that work with the body's slower evening rhythm.

Why Dinner Carbohydrates Require a Different Approach

As the day progresses, the body's ability to process large carbohydrate loads can change. Physical activity is typically lower in the evening, and digestion begins to slow as the body prepares for rest.

Carbohydrates consumed at dinner are therefore more likely to remain in circulation longer if portions are large or if meals lack balance. This can lead to elevated blood sugar levels that persist into the night.

Understanding this shift helps explain why dinner carbohydrates feel more impactful than those eaten earlier in the day.

Choosing Carbohydrates That Support the Evening

Not all carbohydrates behave the same way. Whole grains, legumes, vegetables, and fiber-rich foods digest more slowly and create a gentler blood sugar response.

Refined carbohydrates, such as white rice, white pasta, and sugary sauces, digest quickly and may cause blood sugar levels to rise more sharply. Choosing higher-fiber options helps reduce this effect.

At dinner, smaller portions of carbohydrates paired with protein and vegetables are often more effective than larger, carb-centered meals.

Pairing for Overnight Stability

Protein plays an important role in evening meals. It slows digestion and supports fullness, reducing the likelihood of late-night hunger. Vegetables add fiber and volume without excessive carbohydrate load.

When carbohydrates are paired with these elements, the overall blood sugar response becomes steadier. This pairing helps the body transition into rest without disruption.

A balanced dinner plate often includes a solid protein source, a generous portion of vegetables, and a moderate amount of carbohydrates. This structure supports both satisfaction and overnight balance.

Avoiding the All-or-Nothing Mindset

One of the most common challenges with dinner carbohydrates is an all-or-nothing approach. Avoiding carbohydrates entirely can lead to feelings of deprivation, while unrestricted intake can disrupt blood sugar balance.

This book encourages a middle path. Including carbohydrates intentionally allows meals to feel complete without overwhelming the body late in the day.

This approach supports consistency and reduces the likelihood of rebound eating or late-night snacking.

Building Confidence Through Routine

As you gain experience with balanced dinner combinations, confidence grows. Certain carbohydrate choices and portion sizes will begin to feel dependable, helping remove uncertainty from evening meals.

The recipes in this book are designed to demonstrate how carbohydrates can be included at dinner without disruption. They offer practical examples of balance in action.

In the next chapter, we will focus on smart dinner shopping, helping you choose ingredients that make balanced evening meals easier to prepare, even on busy nights.

Chapter 4

Smart Dinner Shopping

Dinner shopping sets the tone for how evenings unfold. When ingredients are chosen with intention, preparing a balanced meal feels simpler and less stressful. When shopping is rushed or unplanned, dinner decisions often become reactive, especially at the end of a long day.

Smart dinner shopping is about creating an environment that supports calm, nourishing evenings.

Shopping With Evenings in Mind

Dinner ingredients should reflect how evenings actually feel. Energy is often lower, time may be limited, and patience can be thin. Choosing ingredients that are easy to prepare helps prevent frustration and last-minute choices.

Proteins such as chicken, fish, lean meats, tofu, and legumes form the foundation of balanced dinners. These foods provide structure and satiety, helping regulate blood sugar levels overnight.

Vegetables should make up a generous portion of dinner shopping. Fresh, frozen, or pre-cut vegetables all offer flexibility and convenience. Having vegetables readily available makes it easier to build meals around them rather than relying on carbohydrate-heavy options.

Navigating Packaged and Prepared Foods

Packaged and prepared foods can be helpful in the evening, but they require careful selection. Many convenience meals contain refined carbohydrates, added sugars, and large portion sizes.

When choosing packaged items, look for options with clear ingredient lists and balanced nutrition. Avoid meals where refined grains or sugars dominate the ingredient list.

Sauces, marinades, and condiments deserve special attention. These items often contain hidden sugars that can significantly affect blood sugar levels. Choosing simple, low-sugar options or preparing basic sauces at home provides greater control.

Choosing Carbohydrates for Dinner

Dinner carbohydrates should be selected with portion and quality in mind. Whole grains, legumes, and starchy vegetables provide carbohydrates that digest more slowly and support steadier blood sugar levels.

Stocking the kitchen with these options makes it easier to include carbohydrates thoughtfully rather than impulsively.

Limiting highly refined carbohydrate products reduces the likelihood of overeating or blood sugar disruption later in the evening.

Planning for Ease and Comfort

Dinner shopping should support ease, not complexity. Choosing ingredients that can be prepared quickly or used across multiple meals helps reduce evening stress.

Buying proteins and vegetables that can be cooked in batches provides flexibility for different dinner combinations throughout the week.

Keeping a short list of dependable dinner staples helps simplify choices and build consistency.

Creating a Supportive Evening Routine

When your kitchen is stocked with appropriate dinner ingredients, the path of least resistance becomes the healthier one. This reduces decision fatigue and supports better habits without relying on willpower.

Over time, dinner shopping becomes more intuitive, and evenings feel more manageable.

In the next chapter, we will focus on preparation strategies that make dinner easier on busy nights, helping you maintain balance even when time is limited.

Chapter 5

Prep Strategies for Busy Evenings

Evenings can be the most challenging time of day for preparing meals. Fatigue, time pressure, and competing responsibilities often make cooking feel like a burden rather than a comfort. For individuals managing Type 2 Diabetes, these pressures can increase the temptation to rely on convenience foods that do not support blood sugar balance.

Simple preparation strategies help reduce this strain and make balanced dinners more achievable.

Preparing Ahead for Smoother Evenings

Preparing components in advance can significantly ease the demands of evening cooking. Cooking proteins ahead of time, such as chicken, fish, or legumes, provides a foundation for quick meals later in the week.

Chopping vegetables in advance or choosing pre-cut options saves time and reduces barriers to healthier choices. When ingredients are ready to use, assembling a balanced dinner becomes far less overwhelming.

Preparing just one or two elements ahead of time can make a noticeable difference on busy nights.

One-Pan and Simple Cooking Methods

Dinner does not need to involve multiple dishes or complicated steps. One-pan meals, sheet-pan dinners, and simple stovetop recipes help minimize cleanup and reduce mental load.

These methods allow proteins, vegetables, and carbohydrates to be cooked together in a balanced way, saving time and effort. Simple seasoning and cooking techniques keep meals flavorful without adding complexity.

This approach supports consistency by making cooking feel manageable.

Using Leftovers Intentionally

Leftovers can be an effective dinner strategy when planned intentionally. Cooking slightly larger portions earlier in the week creates ready-to-eat meals for nights when time or energy is limited.

The key is balance. Leftover meals should include protein, vegetables, and controlled carbohydrate portions. When leftovers are well-balanced, they support blood sugar stability just as effectively as freshly prepared meals.

Storing leftovers in clear containers helps make them visible and accessible.

Quick Solutions for Low-Energy Nights

Not every evening allows for cooking, and that is normal. Keeping a few reliable, quick options on hand helps prevent skipped dinners or impulsive choices.

Frozen vegetables, pre-cooked proteins, and simple pantry staples can be combined quickly to create balanced meals. These options support flexibility without sacrificing nutrition.

Having these backups reduces stress and helps maintain consistency.

Creating an Evening Cooking Rhythm

Consistency at dinner helps reinforce healthy patterns. Establishing a loose evening routine, such as cooking at a similar time or using familiar recipes, reduces decision fatigue.

This routine does not need to be rigid. It simply provides structure that supports follow-through.

In the next chapter, we will focus on portion awareness at dinner, helping you enjoy satisfying meals without feeling overly full or uncomfortable later in the evening.

Chapter 6

Portion Awareness for Comfortable Evenings

Portion size at dinner has a direct impact on how you feel during the evening and how your body responds overnight. Even nutritious foods can cause discomfort or disrupt blood sugar balance when portions are larger than the body needs.

Portion awareness at dinner is not about restriction. It is about finding the amount that feels satisfying without causing heaviness, discomfort, or late-night blood sugar challenges.

Why Dinner Portions Matter More at Night

As the day comes to a close, digestion naturally slows. Large meals require more energy to process, which can interfere with relaxation and sleep.

For individuals managing Type 2 Diabetes, large portions of carbohydrates at dinner can lead to prolonged blood sugar elevations. These elevations may continue into the night, affecting sleep quality and morning blood sugar levels.

Balanced portions help support a smoother transition into rest.

Recognizing Comfortable Dinner Portions

A comfortable dinner portion often looks slightly smaller than a lunch portion. Protein and vegetables should make up the majority of the meal, providing fullness and nourishment without excessive carbohydrate load.

Carbohydrates should be present but controlled. Smaller portions paired with protein and fiber help prevent spikes and support overnight stability.

Eating slowly and without distraction can also improve portion awareness. Taking time to notice fullness cues helps prevent overeating.

Common Evening Portion Challenges

Evenings often bring emotional eating triggers. Stress, fatigue, and the desire for comfort can lead to larger portions than intended.

Second helpings, late-night snacking, and oversized servings are common challenges. Recognizing these patterns allows for gentle adjustments rather than self-criticism.

Addressing portion size does not mean eliminating enjoyment. It means creating balance that feels supportive.

Adjusting Portions for Better Evenings

If dinner leaves you feeling overly full, restless, or uncomfortable, it may be a sign that portions need adjustment. Reducing carbohydrate portions slightly or increasing vegetables can often improve outcomes.

On days with higher activity levels, slightly larger portions may feel appropriate. Flexibility allows meals to adapt to your needs without losing structure.

Building a Calm Evening Routine

Over time, portion awareness becomes intuitive. As you learn what feels comfortable in the evening, dinner becomes less stressful and more enjoyable.

The recipes in this book are designed with portion awareness in mind, helping remove guesswork and support comfortable evenings.

In the next section, we will transition into the dinner recipes, where these principles come together in practical, satisfying meals designed for the end of the day.

Bringing the Day to a Close

The guidance you have explored in this section is meant to help you approach dinner with confidence rather than hesitation. Understanding how Type 2 Diabetes interacts with evening meals, learning to include carbohydrates thoughtfully, and developing practical habits around shopping, preparation, and portion awareness all serve one purpose. . . to help you end the day feeling supported and at ease.

Now it is time to bring these principles to the table.

The dinner recipes that follow are designed to be comforting, balanced, and realistic for everyday evenings. Each meal emphasizes thoughtful combinations of protein, vegetables, and controlled carbohydrates to support steady blood sugar levels without sacrificing satisfaction.

You do not need to prepare every recipe or follow them in order. Choose meals that fit your schedule, your energy level, and your preferences. Some evenings may call for simple, familiar dishes, while others may allow time for something new. Both are supported here.

As you work through the recipes, pay attention to how different meals affect your comfort, sleep, and overall sense of balance. Use that awareness to guide future choices, making adjustments that feel sustainable.

This section is not about rigid rules or perfect meals. It is about creating dinners that help you unwind, nourish your body, and prepare for rest.

Let these recipes support calmer evenings and more confident mornings ahead.

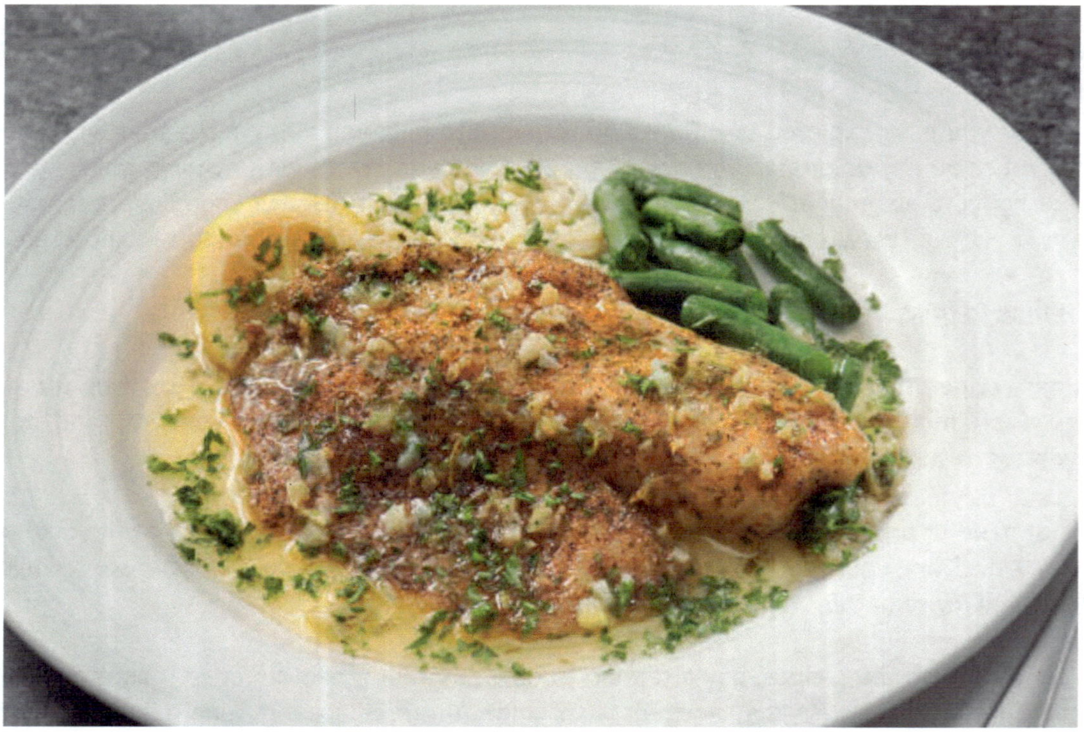

1. Lemon Garlic Grilled Tilapia with Roasted Asparagus

Prep.Time: 15 min

Cook Time: 10-12 min

Serving: 2

Beverage pairing: Iced Tea

Ingredients:

- 2 tilapia fillets
- 2 cloves garlic, minced
- 1 lemon, juiced and zested
- 1 tablespoon olive oil
- Salt and pepper to taste
- 1 bunch asparagus, trimmed
- Cooking spray

Preparation:

1. Preheat the grill to medium-high heat.
2. In a small bowl, mix minced garlic, lemon juice, lemon zest, olive oil, salt, and pepper.
3. Place tilapia fillets in a shallow dish and pour the lemon garlic marinade over them. Allow them to marinate for 15-20 minutes.
4. Meanwhile, preheat the oven to 400°F (200°C). Place the trimmed asparagus on a baking sheet, spray with cooking spray, and sprinkle with salt and pepper. Roast in the oven for 10-12 minutes, or until tender.
5. Grill the marinated tilapia fillets for 3-4 minutes per side, or until cooked through and flaky.
6. Serve the grilled tilapia alongside the roasted asparagus.

Nutrition Facts (per serving):

- Calories: 250
- Carbs: 9g
- Protein: 35g
- Fat: 8g

2. Cauliflower and Edamame Stir-Fry with Sesame Ginger Sauce

Prep.Time: 10 min

Cook Time: 10 min

Serving: 2

Beverage pairing: Mint Water

Ingredients:

- 1 small head cauliflower, chopped into florets
- 1 cup frozen edamame, shelled
- 2 tablespoons low-sodium soy sauce
- 1 tablespoon sesame oil
- 1 teaspoon grated ginger
- 2 cloves garlic, minced
- 1 tablespoon rice vinegar
- 1 tablespoon sesame seeds
- Cooking spray

Preparation:

1. Steam the cauliflower florets and edamame until tender-crisp, about 5-7 minutes.
2. In a small bowl, whisk together soy sauce, sesame oil, grated ginger, minced garlic, and rice vinegar to make the sauce.
3. Heat a non-stick skillet over medium heat and lightly spray with cooking spray.
4. Add steamed cauliflower and edamame to the skillet and pour the sesame ginger sauce over them.
5. Stir-fry for 2-3 minutes until everything is well-coated and heated through.
6. Sprinkle with sesame seeds before serving.

Nutrition Facts (per serving):

- Calories: 180
- Carbs: 14g
- Protein: 10g
- Fat: 10g

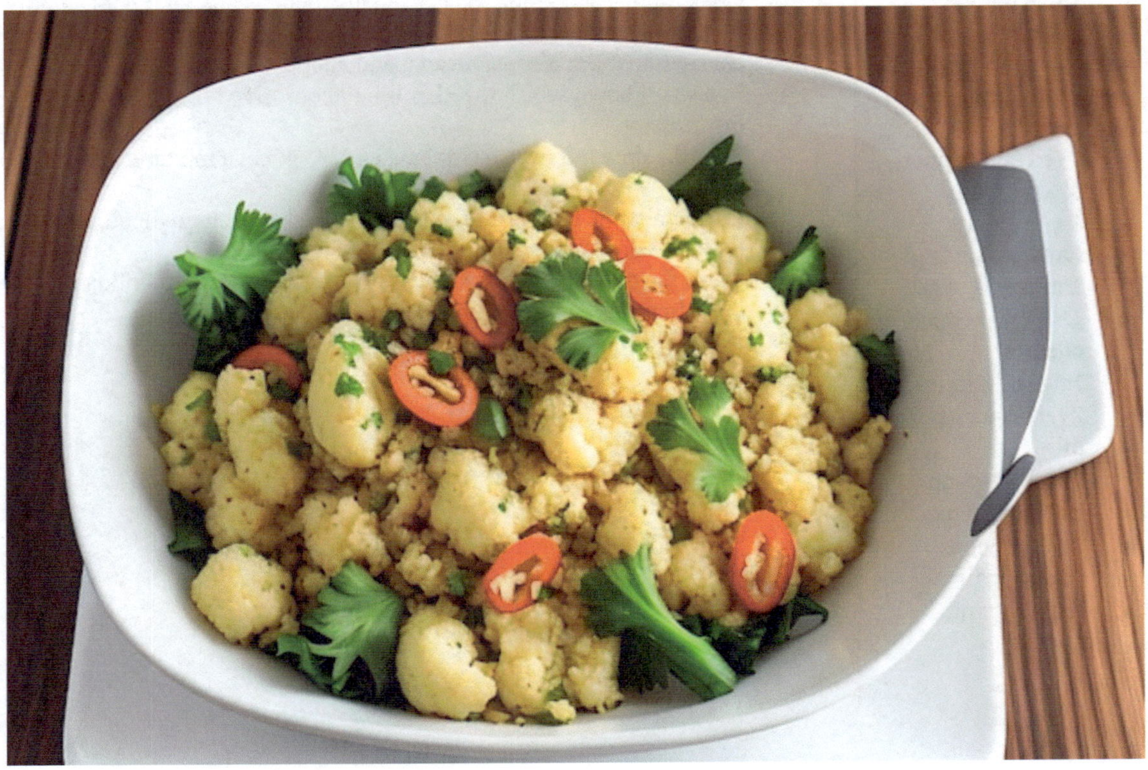

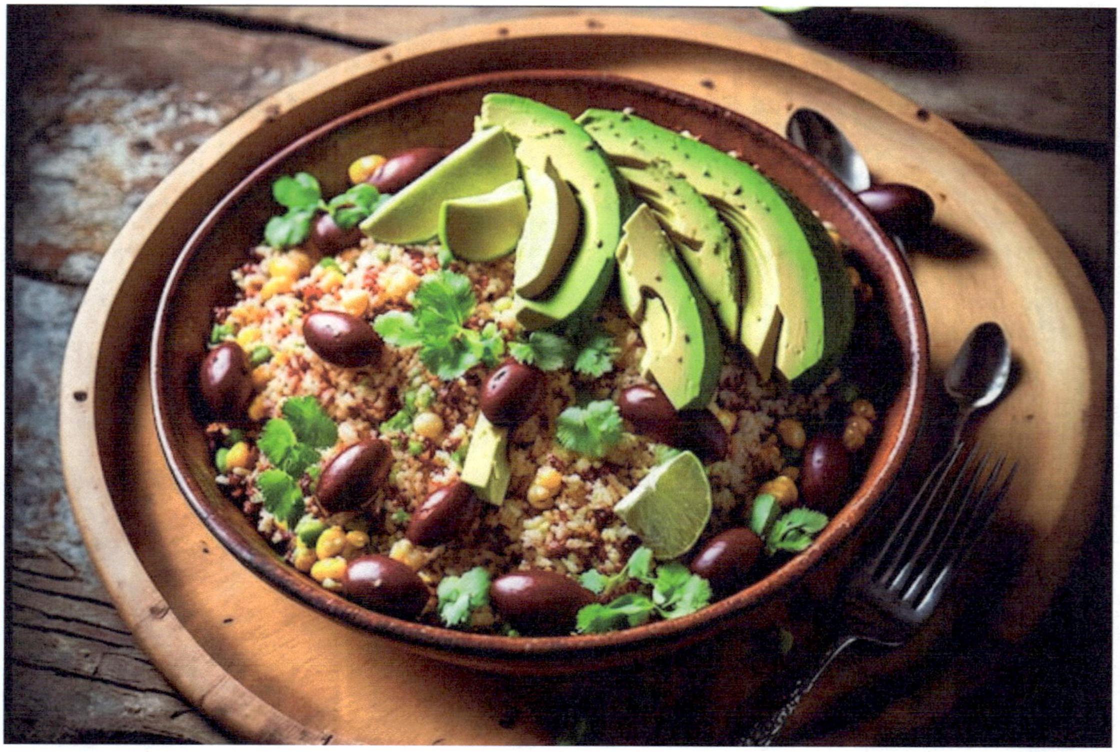

3. Quinoa and Black Bean Bowl with Avocado Lime Dressing

Prep.Time: 20 min

Cook Time: 15 min

Serving: 4

Beverage pairing: Herbal Tea

Ingredients:

- 1 cup quinoa, rinsed
- 1 can (15 oz) black beans, drained and rinsed
- 1 red bell pepper, diced
- 1 cup cherry tomatoes, halved
- 1 avocado, diced
- 1/4 cup chopped cilantro
- Juice of 2 limes
- 2 tablespoons olive oil
- 1 ripe avocado
- Juice of 1 lime
- 2 tablespoons Greek yogurt
- 1 clove garlic, minced

Preparation:

1. Cook quinoa according to package instructions and let it cool slightly.
2. In a large bowl, combine cooked quinoa, black beans, diced bell pepper, cherry tomatoes, diced avocado, and chopped cilantro.
3. In a small bowl, whisk together lime juice, olive oil, salt, and pepper to make the dressing.
4. Pour the dressing over the quinoa and black bean mixture, and toss gently to coat.
5. In a blender or food processor, blend together all ingredients for the avocado lime dressing until smooth.
6. Serve the quinoa and black bean mixture topped with a dollop of avocado lime dressing.

Nutrition Facts (per serving):

- Calories: 380
- Carbs: 46g
- Protein: 11g
- Fat: 18g

4. Grilled Chicken and Vegetable Lettuce Wraps with Cilantro Lime Sauce

Prep.Time: 15 min

Cook Time: 15 min

Serving: 4

Beverage pairing: Lemonade

Ingredients:

- 2 boneless, skinless chicken breasts
- 1 red bell pepper, thinly sliced
- 1 yellow bell pepper, thinly sliced
- 1 zucchini, thinly sliced
- 1 tablespoon olive oil
- 1 head butter lettuce, leaves separated
- 1/4 cup Greek yogurt
- Juice of 1 lime
- 2 tablespoons chopped cilantro
- 1 clove garlic, minced

Preparation:

1. Preheat the grill to medium-high heat.
2. Season chicken breasts with salt and pepper and grill for 6-8 minutes per side, or until cooked through.
3. In a bowl, toss sliced bell peppers and zucchini with olive oil, salt, and pepper. Grill the vegetables for 3-4 minutes until tender-crisp.
4. Once cooked, thinly slice the grilled chicken breasts.
5. In a small bowl, mix together Greek yogurt, lime juice, chopped cilantro, minced garlic, salt, and pepper to make the cilantro lime sauce.
6. To assemble the lettuce wraps, place a few slices of grilled chicken and grilled vegetables onto each lettuce leaf. Drizzle with cilantro lime sauce.
7. Serve immediately.

Nutrition Facts (per serving):

- Calories: 220
- Carbs: 8g
- Protein: 28g
- Fat: 8g

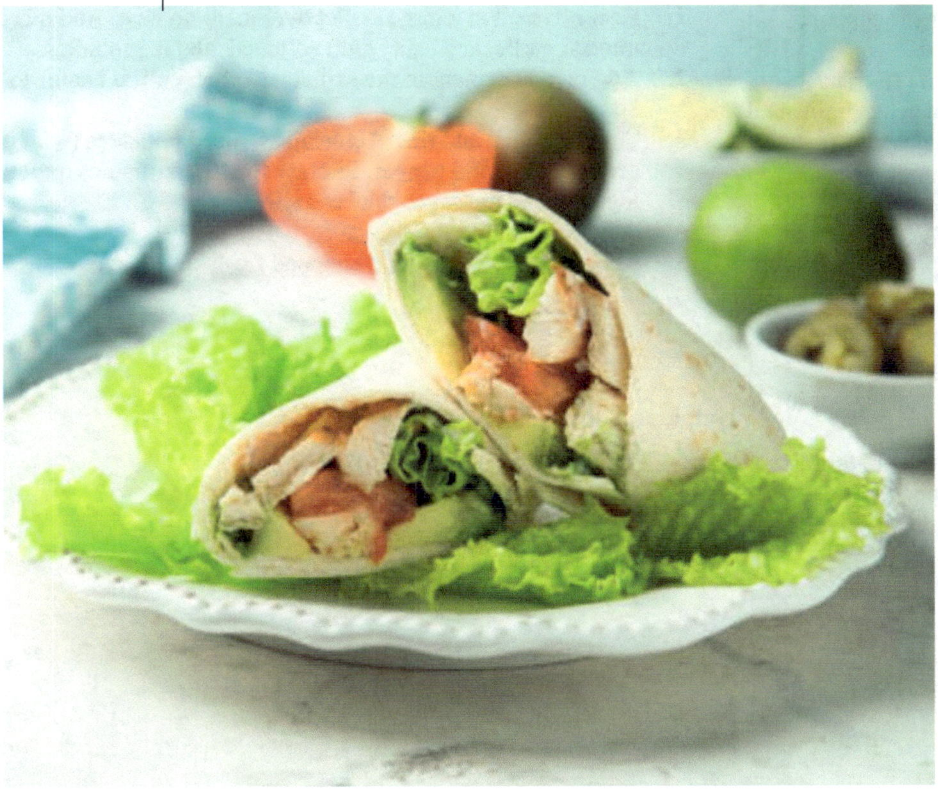

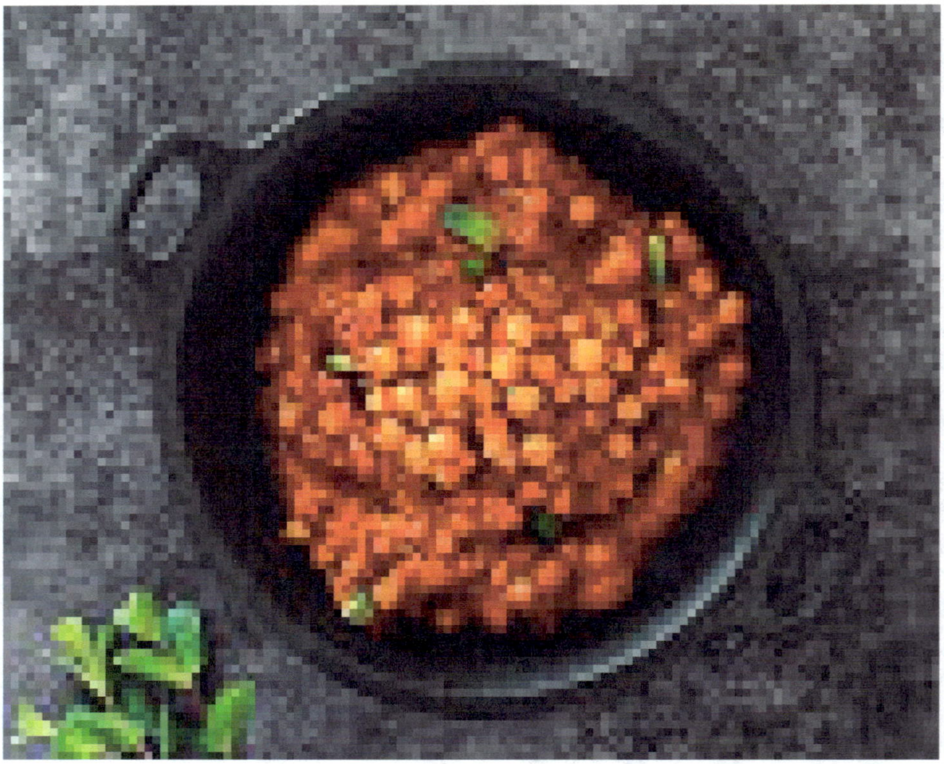

5. Eggplant and Chickpea Ratatouille with Basil

Prep.Time: 10 min

Cook Time: 25 min

Serving: 4

Beverage pairing: Herbal Tea

Ingredients:

- 1 large eggplant, diced
- 1 can (15 oz) chickpeas, drained and rinsed
- 1 onion, diced
- 2 cloves garlic, minced
- 1 can (14 oz) diced tomatoes
- 1 teaspoon dried oregano
- Salt and pepper to taste
- Fresh basil leaves, chopped, for garnish

Preparation:

1. Heat olive oil in a large skillet over medium heat. Add diced onion and minced garlic, and sauté until softened, about 5 minutes.
2. Add diced eggplant to the skillet and cook until it begins to soften, about 8-10 minutes.
3. Stir in drained and rinsed chickpeas, diced tomatoes (with juices), dried oregano, salt, and pepper. Simmer for 10-15 minutes until the flavors meld together and the sauce thickens slightly.
4. Adjust seasoning if necessary.
5. Serve hot, garnished with chopped fresh basil leaves.

Nutrition Facts (per serving):

- Calories: 220
- Carbs: 38g
- Protein: 9g
- Fat: 4g

6. Shrimp and Broccoli Zoodle Alfredo

Prep.Time: 20 min

Cook Time: 15 min

Serving: 4

Beverage pairing: Lemonade

Ingredients:

- 1 pound shrimp, peeled and deveined
- 2 tablespoons olive oil
- 4 cloves garlic, minced
- 1 head broccoli, cut into florets
- 2 large zucchinis, spiralized into noodles
- 1 cup unsweetened almond milk
- 1/4 cup grated Parmesan cheese
- Salt and pepper to taste
- Fresh parsley for garnish

Preparation:

1. In a large skillet, heat olive oil over medium heat. Add minced garlic and cook until fragrant, about 1 minute.
2. Add shrimp to the skillet and cook until pink and cooked through, about 3-4 minutes per side. Remove shrimp from skillet and set aside.
3. In the same skillet, add broccoli florets and cook until tender-crisp, about 5 minutes.
4. Add zucchini noodles to the skillet and cook for an additional 2-3 minutes, until heated through but still firm.
5. Pour unsweetened almond milk into the skillet and stir in grated Parmesan cheese. Cook until the sauce thickens slightly, about 2-3 minutes.
6. Season with salt and pepper to taste.
7. Return cooked shrimp to the skillet and toss everything together until well combined.
8. Serve hot, garnished with fresh parsley.

Nutrition Facts (per serving):

- Calories: 280
- Carbs: 10g
- Protein: 28g
- Fat: 15g

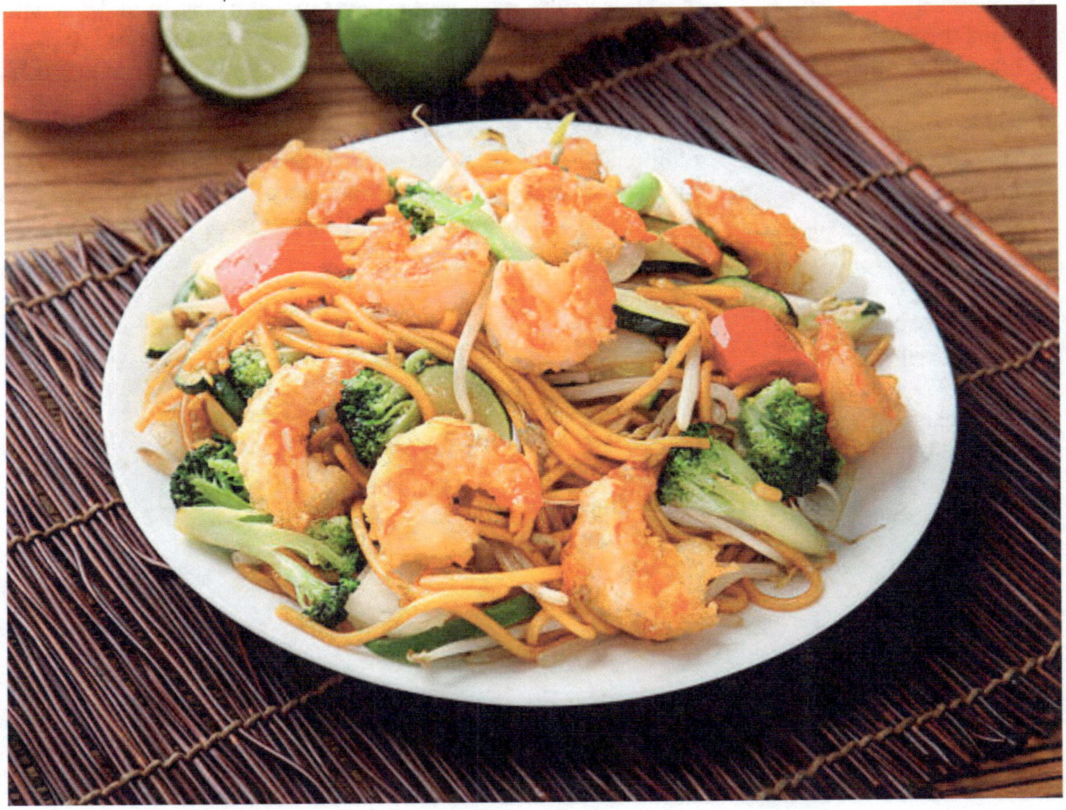

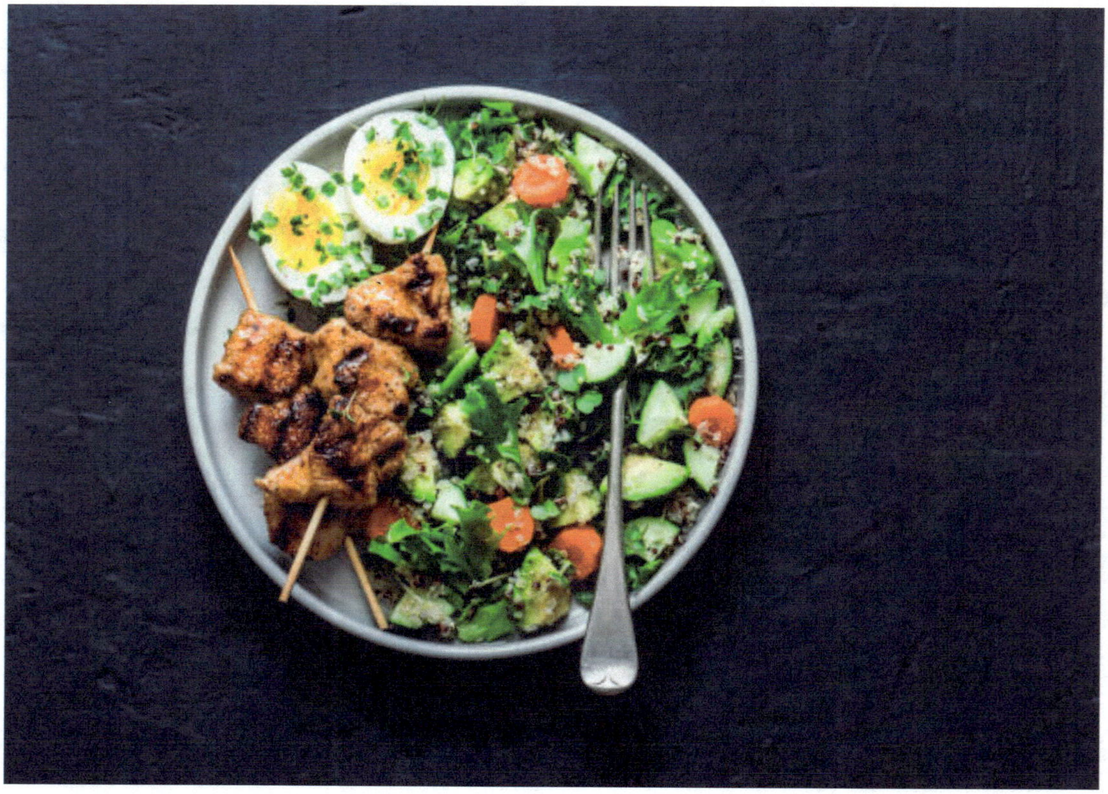

7. Mediterranean Turkey and Quinoa Skillet

Prep.Time: 15 min

Cook Time: 20 min

Serving: 4

Beverage pairing: Herbal Tea

Ingredients:

- 1 pound lean ground turkey
- 1 tablespoon olive oil
- 1 onion, diced
- 2 cloves garlic, minced
- 1 red bell pepper, diced
- 1 cup cherry tomatoes, halved
- 1 cup cooked quinoa
- 1/4 cup chopped Kalamata olives
- 2 tablespoons chopped fresh parsley
- Juice of 1 lemon
- Salt and pepper to taste

Preparation:

1. In a large skillet, heat olive oil over medium heat. Add diced onion and minced garlic, and sauté until softened, about 5 minutes.
2. Add ground turkey to the skillet and cook until browned and cooked through, breaking it up with a spoon as it cooks.
3. Stir in diced bell pepper and halved cherry tomatoes, and cook for an additional 3-4 minutes until vegetables are tender.
4. Add cooked quinoa, chopped Kalamata olives, chopped fresh parsley, and lemon juice to the skillet. Stir well to combine.
5. Season with salt and pepper to taste.
6. Serve hot.

Nutrition Facts (per serving):

- Calories: 320
- Carbs: 20g
- Protein: 26g
- Fat: 14g

8. Cabbage and Carrot Noodle Salad with Turmeric Tahini Dressing

Prep.Time: 15 min

Cook Time: 0 min

Serving: 4

Beverage pairing: Green Tea

Ingredients:

- 1/2 small cabbage, thinly sliced
- 2 large carrots, spiralized into noodles
- 1/4 cup tahini
- 2 tablespoons lemon juice
- 1 tablespoon olive oil
- 1 teaspoon ground turmeric
- 1 clove garlic, minced
- Salt and pepper to taste
- Sesame seeds for garnish

Preparation:

1. In a large bowl, combine thinly sliced cabbage and carrot noodles.
2. In a small bowl, whisk together tahini, lemon juice, olive oil, ground turmeric, minced garlic, salt, and pepper to make the dressing.
3. Pour the dressing over the cabbage and carrot noodles, and toss until well coated.
4. Garnish with sesame seeds before serving.

Nutrition Facts (per serving):

- Calories: 180
- Carbs: 15g
- Protein: 5g
- Fat: 12g

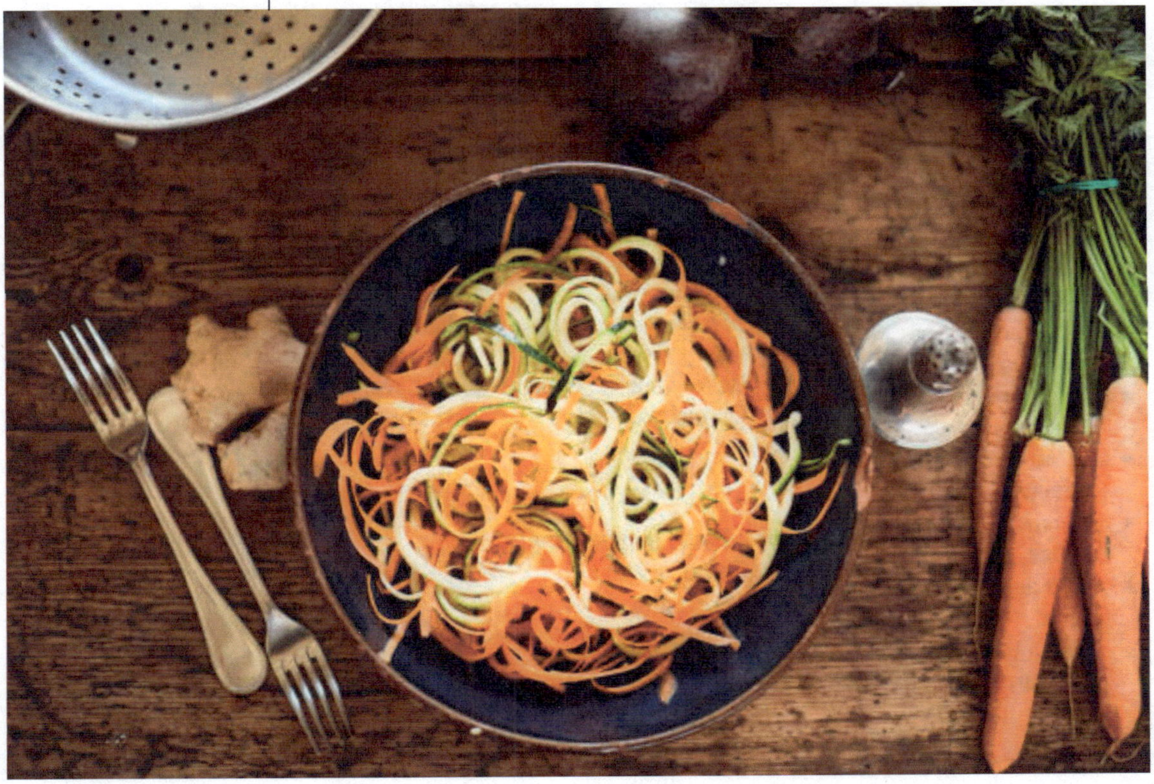

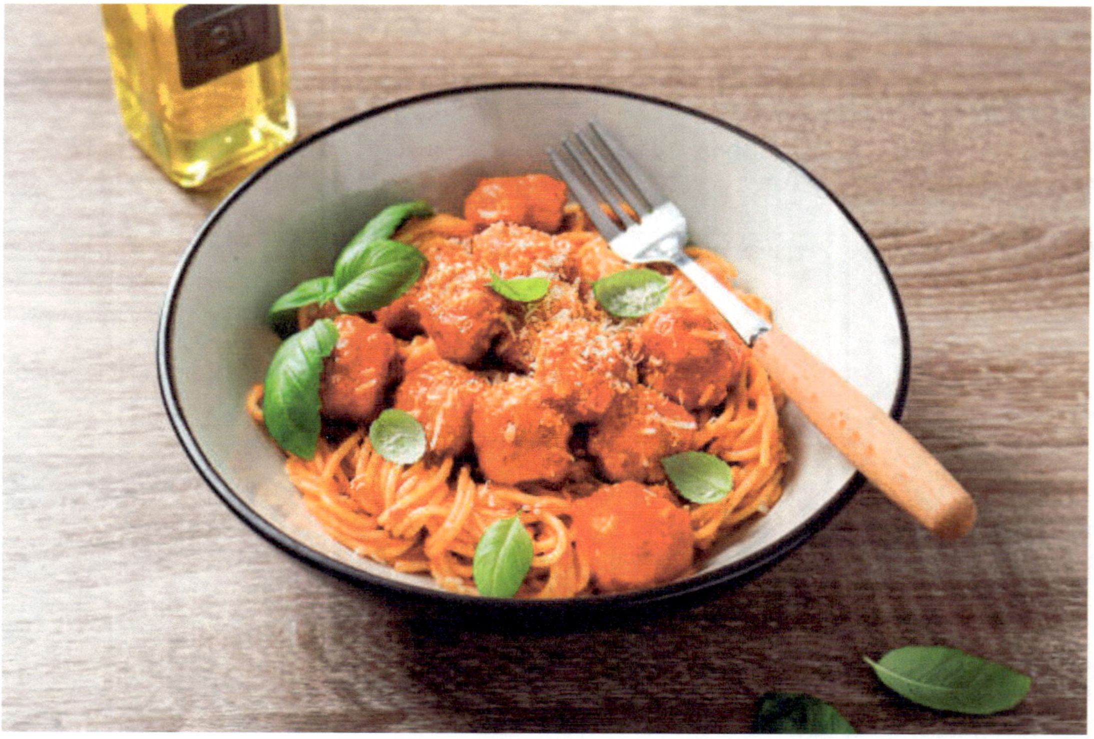

9. Spaghetti Squash and Turkey Meatball Casserole

Prep.Time: 20 min | **Cook Time:** 60 min | **Serving:** 4 | **Beverage pairing:** Herbal Tea

Ingredients:

- 1 large spaghetti squash, halved and seeds removed
- 1 pound lean ground turkey
- 1/4 cup almond flour
- 1 egg
- 1/4 cup grated Parmesan cheese
- 1 teaspoon dried oregano
- 1 teaspoon dried basil
- 1 can (14 oz) diced tomatoes, drained
- 1 cup marinara sauce
- Salt and pepper to taste
- Fresh basil leaves for garnish

Preparation:

1. Preheat oven to 400°F (200°C).
2. Place spaghetti squash halves cut side down on a baking sheet. Bake in the preheated oven for 30-40 minutes, or until squash is tender.
3. In a large bowl, combine ground turkey, almond flour, egg, grated Parmesan cheese, dried oregano, dried basil, salt, and pepper. Mix until well combined, then shape into meatballs.
4. Heat olive oil in a skillet over medium heat. Add turkey meatballs and cook until browned on all sides, about 5-7 minutes.
5. Remove spaghetti squash from the oven and use a fork to scrape the flesh into "noodles".
6. In a baking dish, layer spaghetti squash noodles, diced tomatoes, cooked turkey meatballs, and marinara sauce.
7. Bake in the oven for 15-20 minutes, or until heated through.
8. Garnish with fresh basil leaves before serving.

Nutrition Facts (per serving):

- Calories: 290
- Carbs: 20g
- Protein: 25g
- Fat: 12g

10. Zucchini Ribbon and Tomato Salad with Balsamic Glaze

Prep.Time: 10 min

Cook Time: 0 min

Serving: 4

Beverage pairing: Green Tea

Ingredients:

- 2 large zucchinis, shaved into ribbons
- 1 cup cherry tomatoes, halved
- 1/4 cup chopped fresh basil
- 2 tablespoons balsamic glaze
- 1 tablespoon olive oil
- Salt and pepper to taste
- Shaved Parmesan cheese for garnish (optional)

Preparation:

1. In a large bowl, combine zucchini ribbons, halved cherry tomatoes, and chopped fresh basil.
2. Drizzle olive oil and balsamic glaze over the salad, and toss until well combined.
3. Season with salt and pepper to taste.
4. Garnish with shaved Parmesan cheese, if desired, before serving.

Nutrition Facts (per serving):

- Calories: 120
- Carbs: 10g
- Protein: 3g
- Fat: 7g

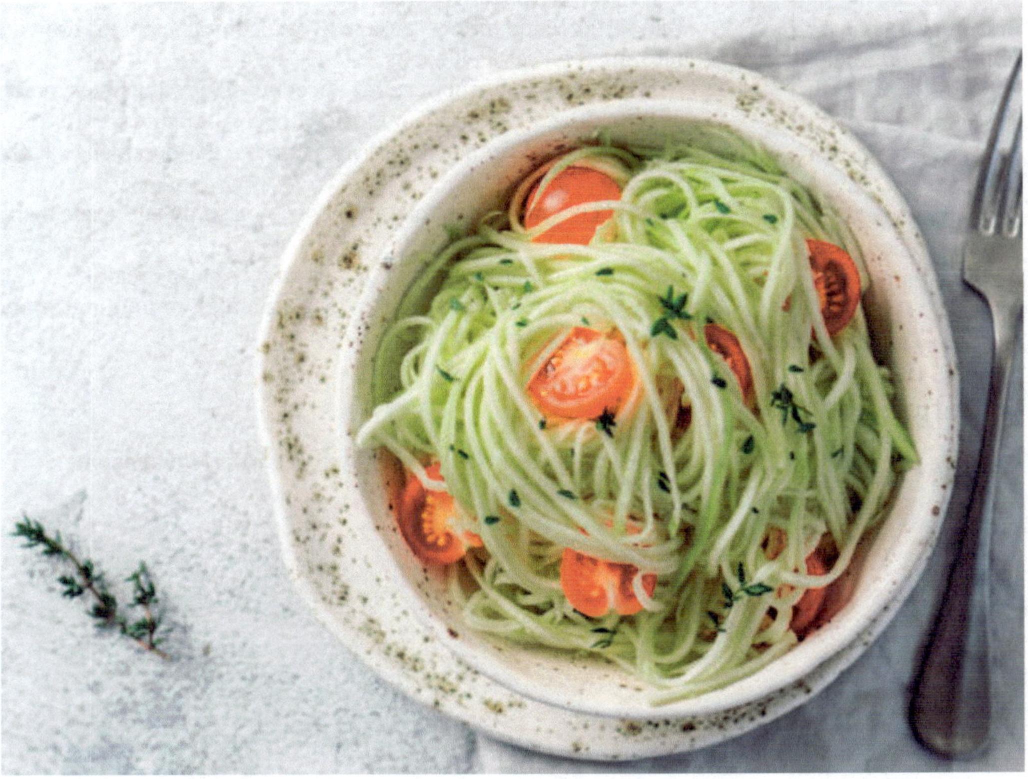

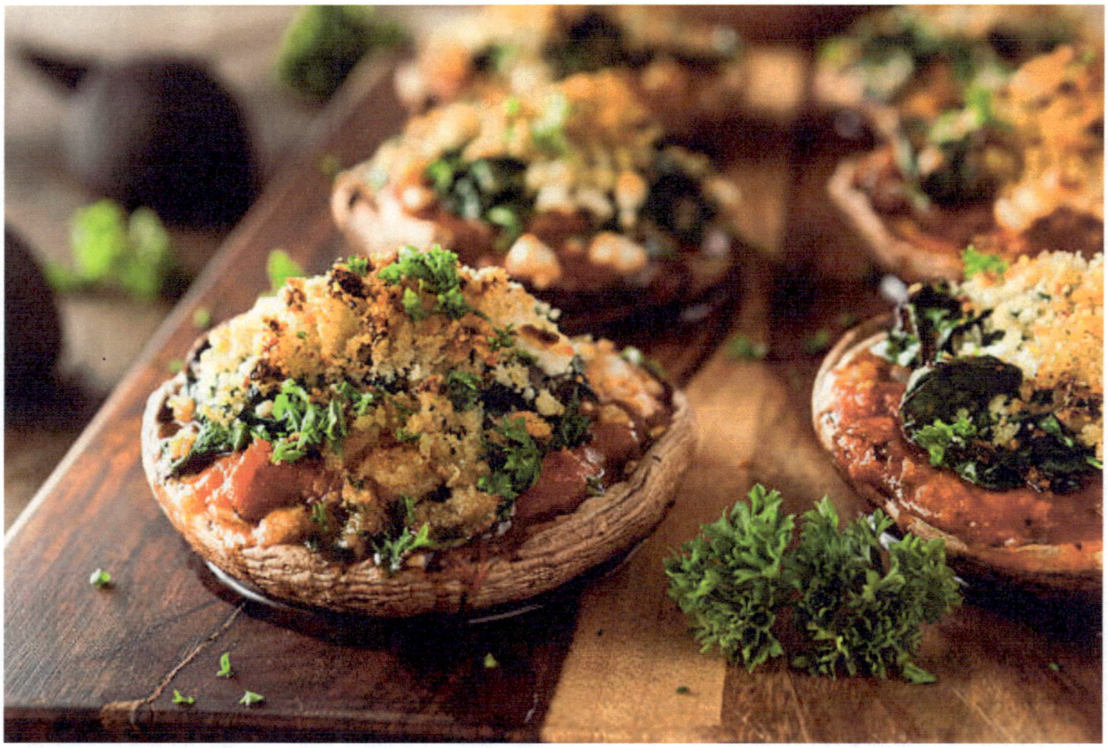

11. Roasted Red Pepper and Turkey Sausage Stuffed Mushrooms

Prep.Time: 15 min

Cook Time: 20 min

Serving: 4

Beverage pairing: Herbal Tea

Ingredients:

- 12 large mushrooms, stems removed and finely chopped
- 1/2 pound turkey sausage, casing removed
- 1/4 cup roasted red peppers, diced
- 2 cloves garlic, minced
- 1/4 cup grated Parmesan cheese
- Salt and pepper to taste
- Cooking spray

Preparation:

1. Preheat oven to 375°F (190°C).
2. In a skillet, cook turkey sausage over medium heat until browned, breaking it into small pieces as it cooks.
3. Add chopped mushroom stems, diced roasted red peppers, and minced garlic to the skillet. Cook until softened, about 3-4 minutes.
4. Remove skillet from heat and stir in grated Parmesan cheese. Season with salt and pepper to taste.
5. Lightly coat mushroom caps with cooking spray and place them on a baking sheet.
6. Stuff each mushroom cap with the turkey sausage mixture.
7. Bake in the preheated oven for 15-20 minutes, or until mushrooms are tender and filling is heated through.

Nutrition Facts (per serving, serving size: 3 stuffed mushrooms):

- Calories: 150
- Carbs: 5g
- Protein: 12g
- Fat: 9g

12. Cauliflower and Broccoli Mash with Garlic Parmesan

Prep.Time: 10 min

Cook Time: 10 min

Serving: 4

Beverage pairing: Herbal Tea

Ingredients:

- 1 small head cauliflower, chopped into florets
- 1 small head broccoli, chopped into florets
- 2 cloves garlic, minced
- 2 tablespoons grated Parmesan cheese
- 1 tablespoon olive oil
- Salt and pepper to taste
- Chopped fresh parsley for garnish (optional)

Preparation:

1. Steam cauliflower and broccoli florets until tender, about 5-7 minutes.
2. In a food processor or blender, combine steamed cauliflower, broccoli, minced garlic, grated Parmesan cheese, olive oil, salt, and pepper. Blend until smooth.
3. Taste and adjust seasoning if necessary.
4. Transfer the mashed cauliflower and broccoli to a serving bowl.
5. Garnish with chopped fresh parsley, if desired, before serving.

Nutrition Facts (per serving):

- Calories: 90
- Carbs: 7g
- Protein: 4g
- Fat: 5g

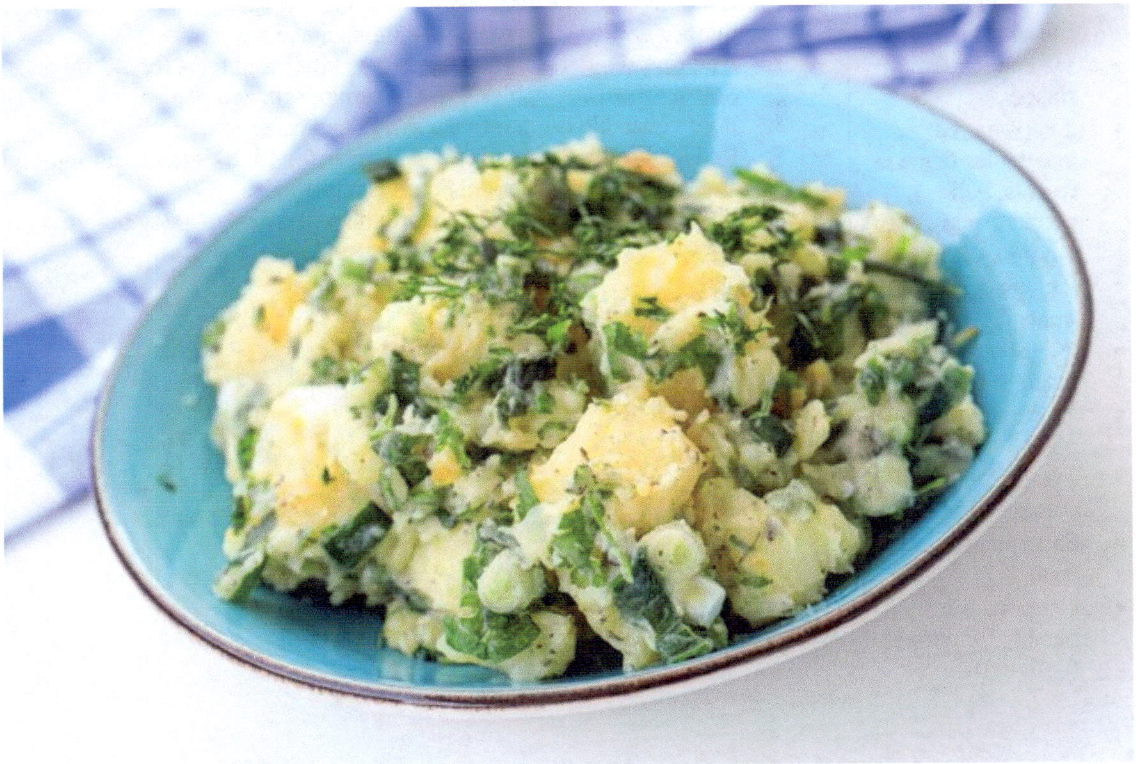

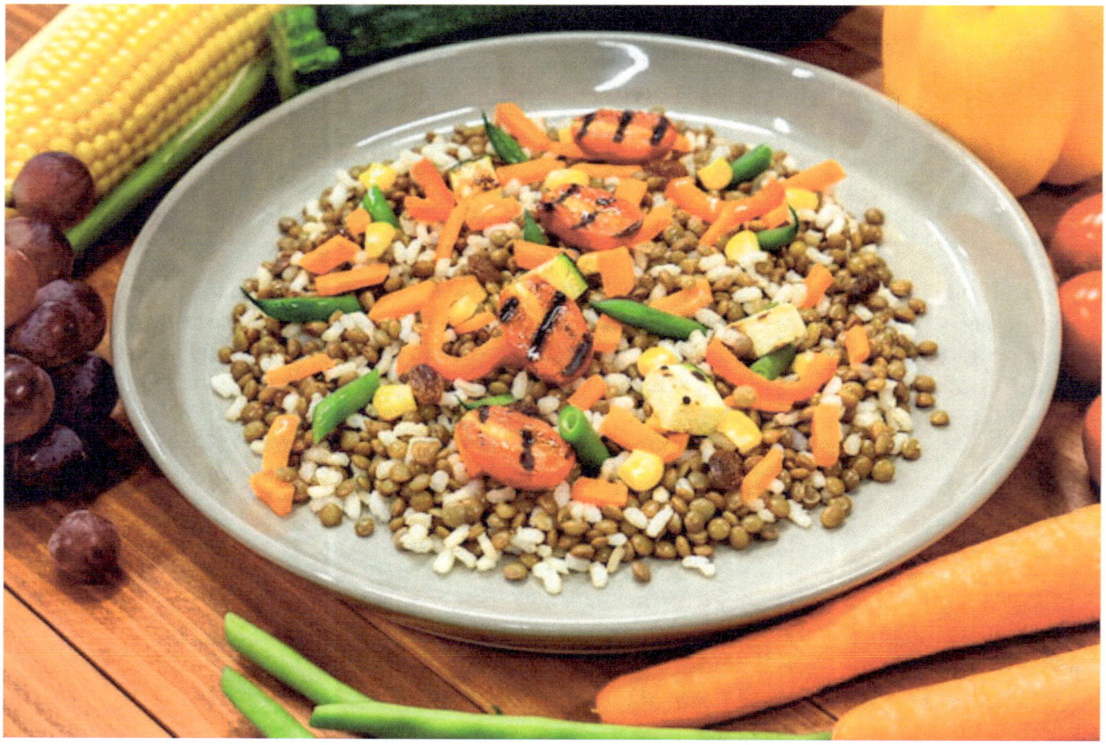

13. Quinoa and Lentil Pilaf with Mixed Vegetables

Prep.Time: 10 min

Cook Time: 25 min

Serving: 4

Beverage pairing: Green Tea

Ingredients:

- 1 cup quinoa, rinsed
- 1/2 cup lentils, rinsed
- 2 cups mixed vegetables (such as carrots, bell peppers, peas, corn)
- 1 onion, diced
- 2 cloves garlic, minced
- 2 cups vegetable broth
- 1 tablespoon olive oil
- 1 teaspoon ground cumin
- Salt and pepper to taste
- Chopped fresh parsley for garnish (optional)

Preparation:

1. Heat olive oil in a large skillet over medium heat. Add diced onion and minced garlic, and sauté until softened, about 5 minutes.
2. Add rinsed quinoa and lentils to the skillet, and toast for 2-3 minutes.
3. Stir in mixed vegetables, ground cumin, salt, and pepper.
4. Pour vegetable broth into the skillet and bring to a boil.
5. Reduce heat to low, cover, and simmer for 15-20 minutes, or until quinoa and lentils are cooked and liquid is absorbed.
6. Fluff with a fork and garnish with chopped fresh parsley before serving.

Nutrition Facts (per serving):

- Calories: 270
- Carbs: 45g
- Protein: 12g
- Fat: 5g

14. Grilled Tofu and Portobello Mushroom Skewers

Prep.Time: 15 min

Cook Time: 10 min

Serving: 4

Beverage pairing: Iced Tea

Ingredients:

- 1 small head cauliflower, chopped into florets
- 1 small head broccoli, chopped into florets
- 2 cloves garlic, minced
- 2 tablespoons grated Parmesan cheese
- 1 tablespoon olive oil
- Salt and pepper to taste
- Chopped fresh parsley for garnish (optional)

Preparation:

1. In a large bowl, whisk together olive oil, balsamic vinegar, minced garlic, dried thyme, salt, and pepper.
2. Add cubed tofu, sliced portobello mushrooms, diced bell peppers, and diced red onion to the bowl. Toss until everything is well coated with the marinade. Let marinate for at least 30 minutes.
3. Preheat grill to medium-high heat.
4. Thread marinated tofu, mushrooms, bell peppers, and red onion onto the soaked wooden skewers.
5. Grill skewers for 8-10 minutes, turning occasionally, until tofu and vegetables are lightly charred and cooked through.
6. Serve hot.

Nutrition Facts (per serving):

- Calories: 220
- Carbs: 12g
- Protein: 14g
- Fat: 14g

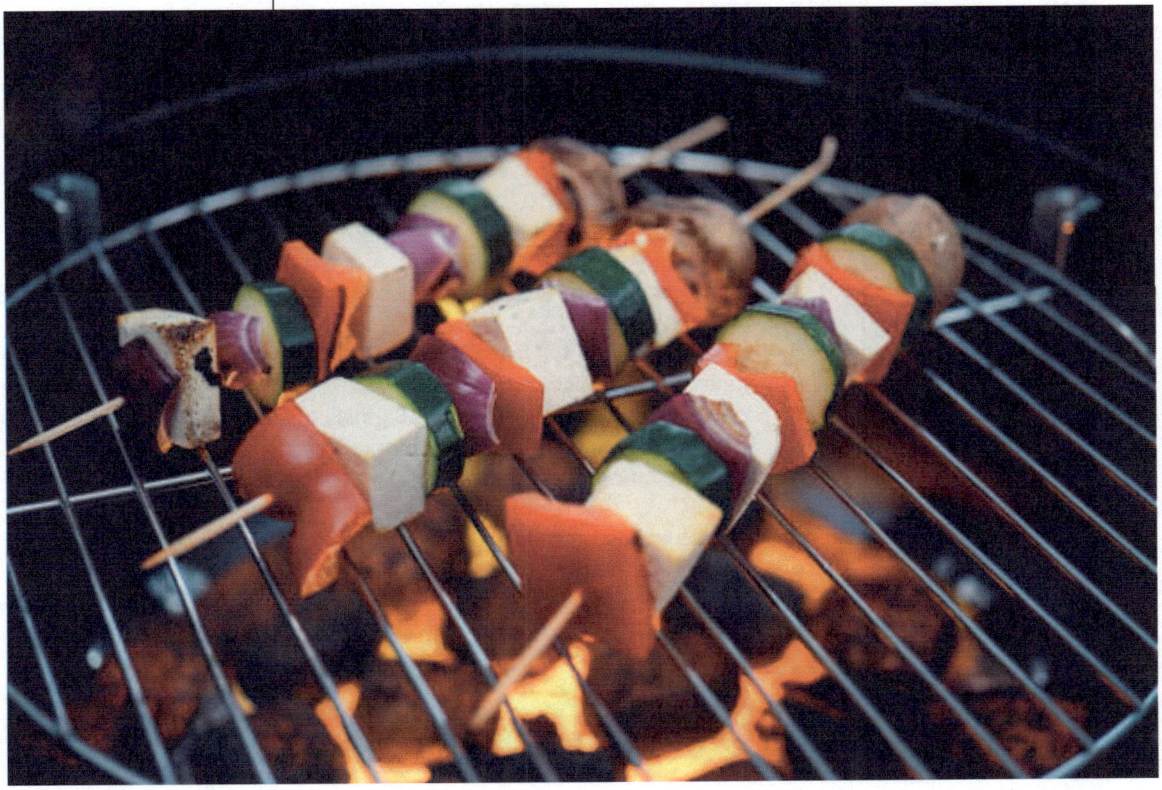

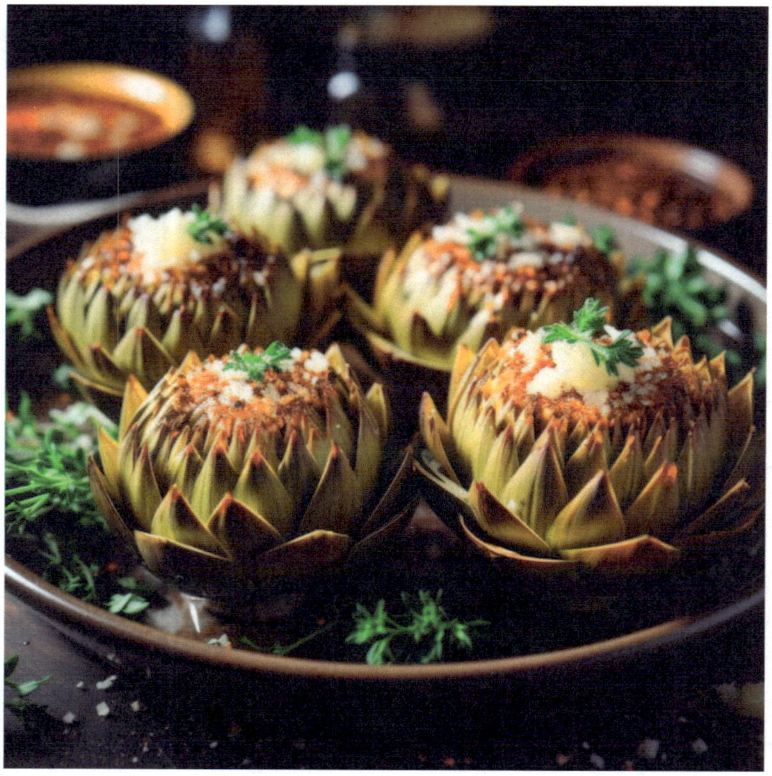

15. Turkey and Spinach Stuffed Artichokes

Prep.Time: 20 min

Cook Time: 45-50 min

Serving: 4

Beverage pairing: Herbal Tea

Ingredients:

- 4 large artichokes
- 1 pound ground turkey
- 2 cups fresh spinach, chopped
- 1/4 cup grated Parmesan cheese
- 2 cloves garlic, minced
- 2 tablespoons olive oil
- 1 tablespoon lemon juice
- Salt and pepper to taste

Preparation:

1. Preheat oven to 375°F (190°C).
2. Trim the stems of the artichokes and remove any tough outer leaves. Cut off the top quarter of each artichoke and use kitchen shears to trim the sharp tips of the remaining leaves.
3. In a skillet, heat olive oil over medium heat. Add minced garlic and cook until fragrant, about 1 minute.
4. Add ground turkey to the skillet and cook until browned, breaking it into small pieces as it cooks.
5. Stir in chopped spinach and cook until wilted.
6. Remove skillet from heat and stir in grated Parmesan cheese, lemon juice, salt, and pepper.
7. Carefully spread the leaves of each artichoke apart and stuff the turkey and spinach mixture between the leaves.
8. Place stuffed artichokes in a baking dish and drizzle with a little olive oil.
9. Cover the baking dish with aluminum foil and bake in the preheated oven for 45-50 minutes, or until the artichokes are tender.

Nutrition Facts (per serving):

- Calories: 280
- Carbs: 20g
- Protein: 24g
- Fat: 12g

16. Lemon Herb Baked Chicken Thighs with Brussels Sprouts

Prep.Time: 15 min | **Cook Time:** 35-40 min | **Serving:** 4 | **Beverage pairing:** Iced Tea

Ingredients:

- 8 bone-in, skin-on chicken thighs
- 1 pound Brussels sprouts, trimmed and halved
- 2 tablespoons olive oil
- 2 cloves garlic, minced
- Zest and juice of 1 lemon
- 1 tablespoon chopped fresh thyme
- Salt and pepper to taste

Preparation:

1. Preheat oven to 400°F (200°C).
2. In a large bowl, toss Brussels sprouts with olive oil, minced garlic, lemon zest, chopped fresh thyme, salt, and pepper.
3. Spread Brussels sprouts out on a baking sheet.
4. Arrange chicken thighs on top of the Brussels sprouts.
5. Drizzle chicken thighs with lemon juice and season with salt and pepper.
6. Bake in the preheated oven for 35-40 minutes, or until chicken is cooked through and Brussels sprouts are tender.
7. Serve hot.

Nutrition Facts (per serving):

- Calories: 380
- Carbs: 10g
- Protein: 32g
- Fat: 24g

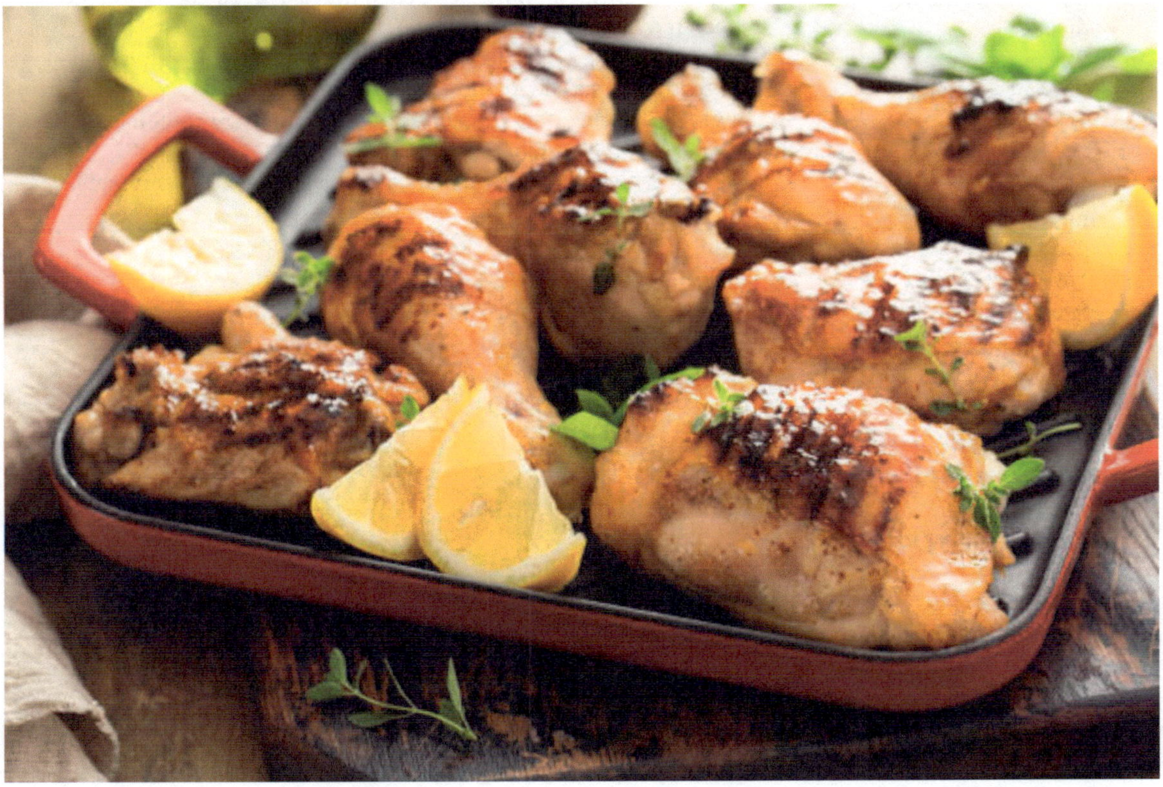

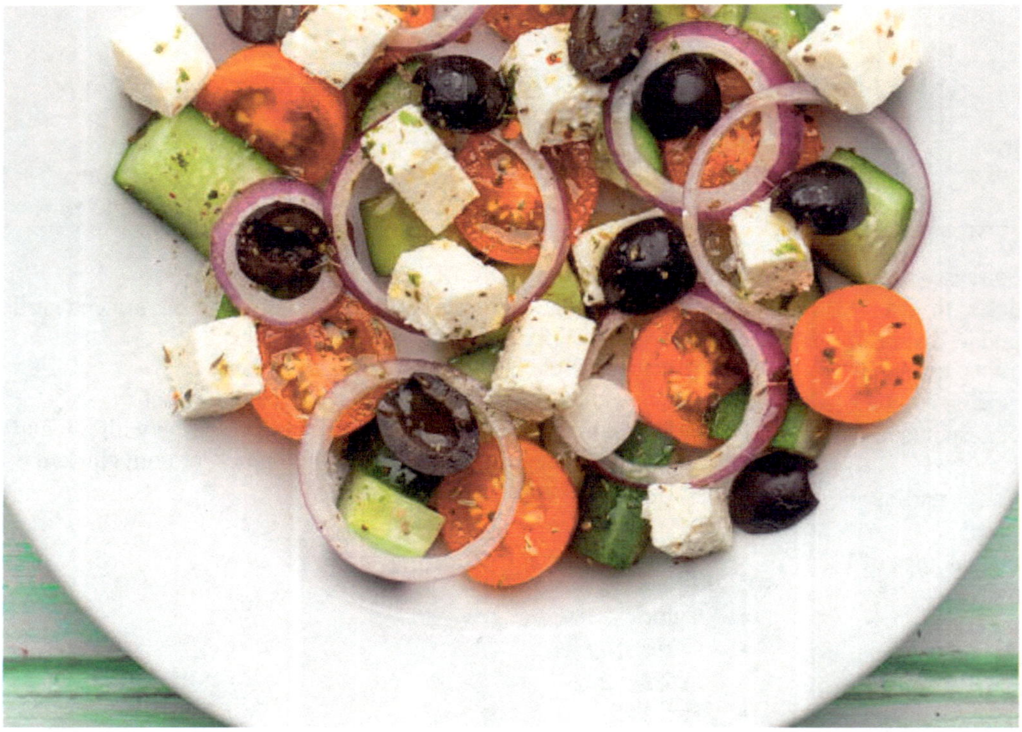

17. Cucumber and Tomato Greek Salad with Feta

Prep.Time: 10 min

Cook Time: 0 min

Serving: 4

Beverage pairing: Herbal Tea

Ingredients:

- 2 large cucumbers, diced
- 2 cups cherry tomatoes, halved
- 1/2 red onion, thinly sliced
- 1/4 cup Kalamata olives, pitted and sliced
- 1/4 cup crumbled feta cheese
- 2 tablespoons extra virgin olive oil
- 1 tablespoon red wine vinegar
- 1 teaspoon dried oregano
- Salt and pepper to taste
- Chopped fresh parsley for garnish (optional)

Preparation:

1. In a large bowl, combine diced cucumbers, halved cherry tomatoes, thinly sliced red onion, and sliced Kalamata olives.
2. In a small bowl, whisk together extra virgin olive oil, red wine vinegar, dried oregano, salt, and pepper to make the dressing.
3. Pour the dressing over the salad and toss until well combined.
4. Sprinkle crumbled feta cheese over the salad.
5. Garnish with chopped fresh parsley, if desired, before serving.

Nutrition Facts (per serving):

- Calories: 120
- Carbs: 8g
- Protein: 3g
- Fat: 9g

18. Baked Cod with Herb Crust and Green Bean Almondine

Prep.Time: 15 min

Cook Time: 15 min

Serving: 4

Beverage pairing: Herbal Tea

Ingredients:

- 4 cod fillets
- 1/4 cup almond meal
- 1 tablespoon chopped fresh parsley
- 1 tablespoon chopped fresh dill
- 1 tablespoon olive oil
- 1 lemon, thinly sliced
- Salt and pepper to taste
- 1 pound green beans, trimmed
- 1/4 cup slivered almonds

Preparation:

1. Preheat oven to 400°F (200°C).
2. In a small bowl, mix together almond meal, chopped fresh parsley, chopped fresh dill, olive oil, salt, and pepper to make the herb crust.
3. Place cod fillets on a baking sheet lined with parchment paper.
4. Spread herb crust evenly over the top of each cod fillet.
5. Arrange lemon slices on top of the herb crust.
6. Bake in the preheated oven for 12-15 minutes, or until cod is cooked through and flakes easily with a fork.
7. While the cod is baking, blanch green beans in boiling water for 2-3 minutes, then drain.
8. In a skillet, toast slivered almonds over medium heat until golden brown.
9. Toss blanched green beans with toasted slivered almonds.
10. Serve baked cod with green bean almondine on the side.

Nutrition Facts (per serving):

- Calories: 250
- Carbs: 10g
- Protein: 30g
- Fat: 12g

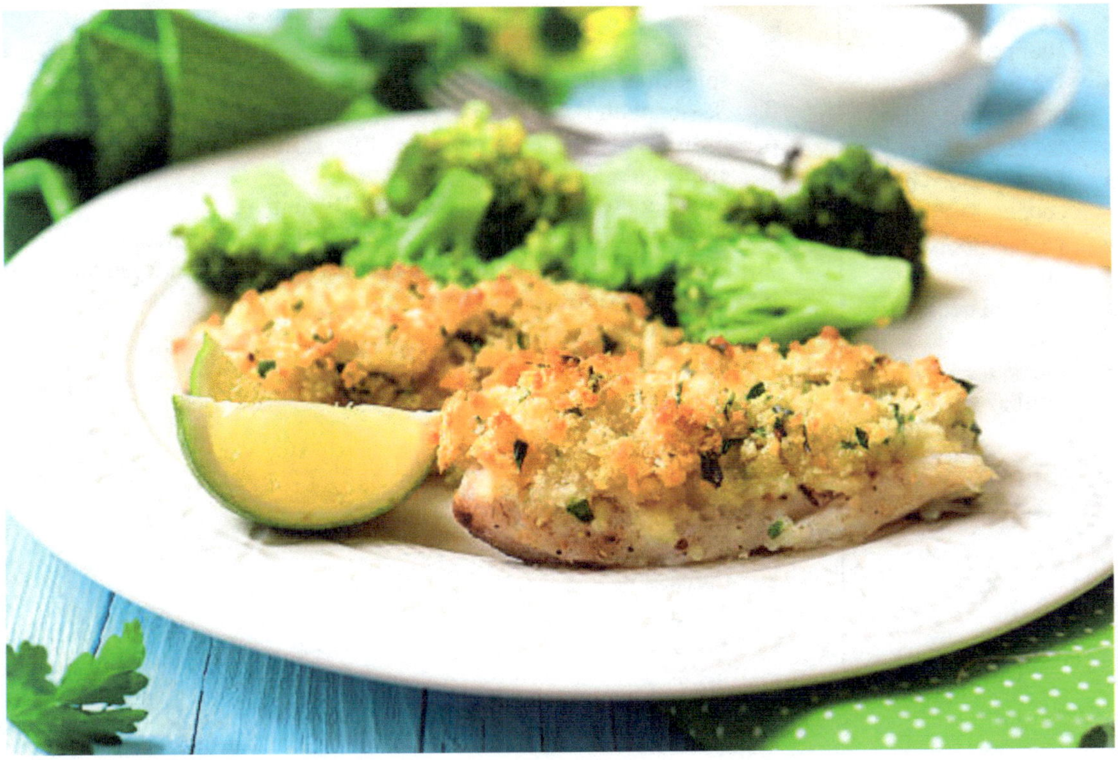

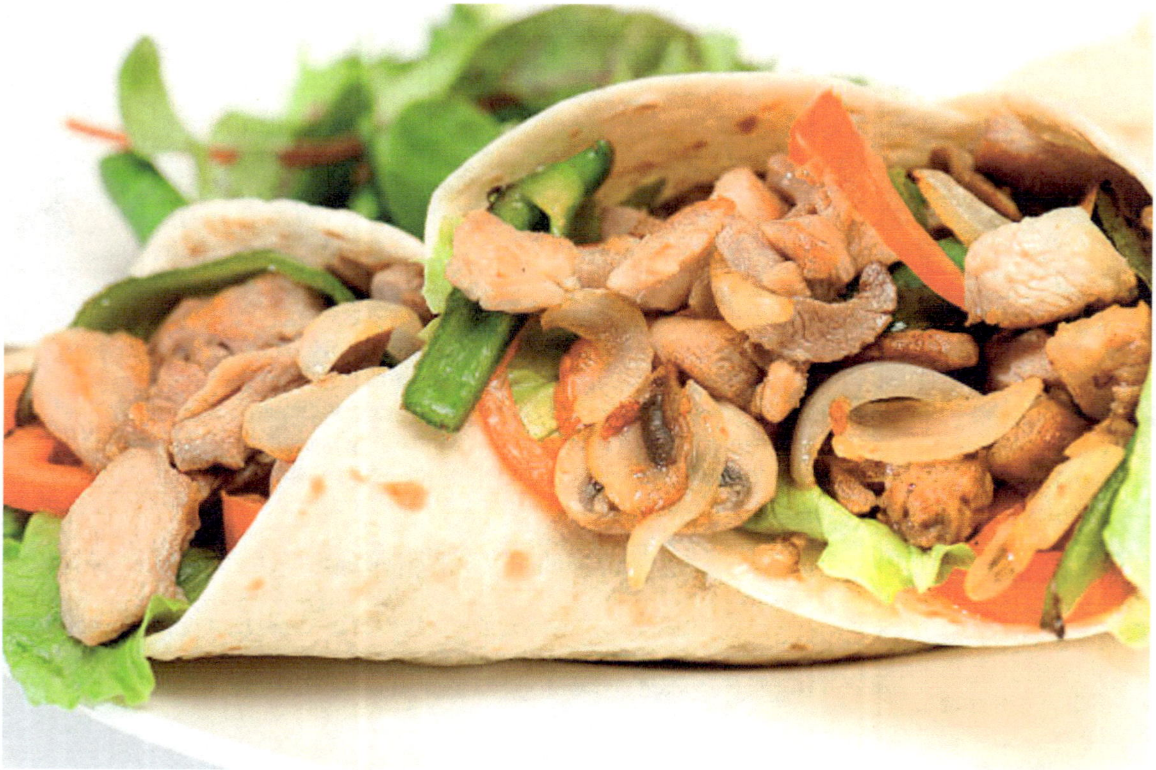

19. Spinach and Mushroom Egg White Breakfast Burrito

Prep.Time: 10 min

Cook Time: 10 min

Serving: 2

Beverage pairing: Green Tea

Ingredients:

- 4 large egg whites
- 1 cup spinach, chopped
- 1/2 cup mushrooms, sliced
- 1/4 cup diced onion
- 1/4 cup diced bell pepper
- 1 tablespoon olive oil
- Salt and pepper to taste
- 2 whole wheat tortillas

Preparation:

1. In a skillet, heat olive oil over medium heat. Add diced onion and sliced mushrooms, and sauté until softened, about 5 minutes.
2. Add chopped spinach and diced bell pepper to the skillet, and cook until spinach is wilted.
3. Season with salt and pepper to taste.
4. Push the vegetables to one side of the skillet and pour egg whites into the empty side.
5. Cook egg whites, stirring occasionally, until set.
6. Warm whole wheat tortillas in the skillet or microwave.
7. Divide cooked egg whites and sautéed vegetables between the tortillas.
8. Roll up the tortillas into burritos.
9. Serve hot.

Nutrition Facts (per serving):

- Calories: 180
- Carbs: 25g
- Protein: 10g
- Fat: 5g

20. Cauliflower and Chickpea Buddha Bowl with Tahini Drizzle

Prep.Time: 15 min | **Cook Time:** 25-30 min | **Serving:** 2 | **Beverage pairing:** Iced Tea

Ingredients:

- 1 small head cauliflower, cut into florets
- 1 can (15 oz) chickpeas, drained and rinsed
- 1 tablespoon olive oil
- 1 teaspoon ground cumin
- 1/2 teaspoon paprika
- 2 cups mixed greens
- 1/4 cup diced cucumber
- 1/4 cup diced tomatoes
- 1/4 cup diced red onion
- 2 tablespoons tahini
- 1 clove garlic, minced

Preparation:

1. Preheat oven to 400°F (200°C).
2. In a large bowl, toss cauliflower florets and chickpeas with olive oil, ground cumin, paprika, salt, and pepper.
3. Spread cauliflower and chickpeas out on a baking sheet and roast in the preheated oven for 25-30 minutes, or until cauliflower is tender and chickpeas are crispy.
4. In a small bowl, whisk together tahini, lemon juice, minced garlic, and water until smooth, adding water as needed to reach desired consistency.
5. To assemble the Buddha bowls, divide mixed greens between bowls and top with roasted cauliflower and chickpeas.
6. Add diced cucumber, diced tomatoes, and diced red onion to each bowl.
7. Drizzle tahini dressing over the top of each bowl.
8. Serve immediately.

Nutrition Facts (per serving):

- Calories: 320
- Carbs: 30g
- Protein: 12g
- Fat: 18g

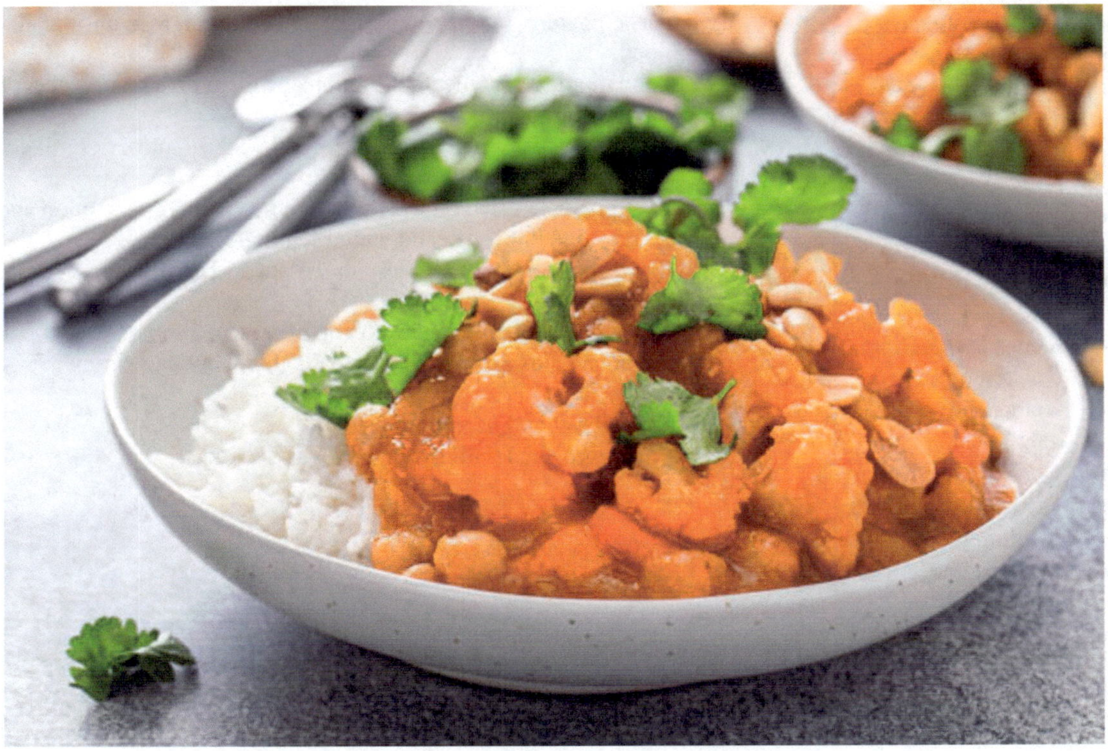

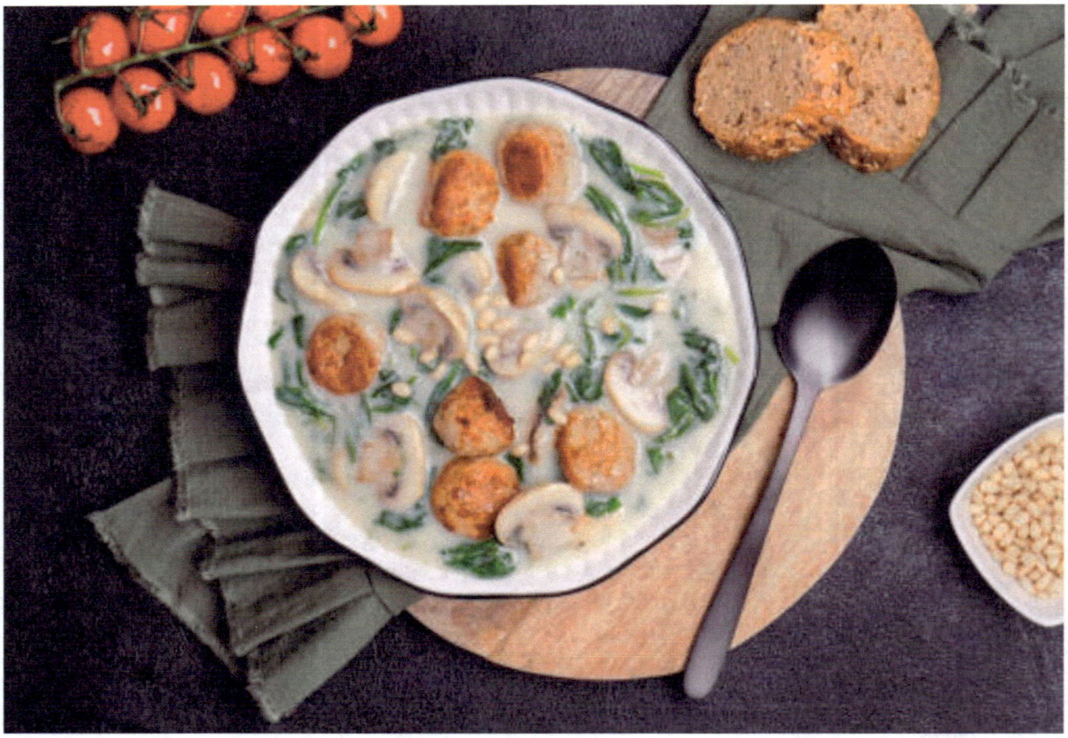

21. Turkey and Kale Meatball Soup

Prep.Time: 20 min

Cook Time: 30 min

Serving: 6

Beverage pairing: Herbal Tea

Ingredients:

- 1 pound lean ground turkey
- 1/2 cup rolled oats
- 1/4 cup grated Parmesan cheese
- 1 egg
- 1 teaspoon garlic powder
- 1 teaspoon onion powder
- Salt and pepper to taste
- 8 cups low-sodium chicken broth
- 2 cups chopped kale
- 1 carrot, diced
- 1 celery stalk, diced
- 1 onion, diced
- 2 cloves garlic, minced
- 1 tablespoon olive oil

Preparation:

1. Preheat oven to 400°F (200°C).
2. In a large bowl, combine ground turkey, rolled oats, grated Parmesan cheese, egg, garlic powder, onion powder, salt, and pepper. Mix until well combined.
3. Shape the mixture into meatballs and place them on a baking sheet lined with parchment paper.
4. Bake meatballs in the preheated oven for 15-20 minutes, or until cooked through.
5. In a large pot, heat olive oil over medium heat. Add diced onion and minced garlic, and sauté until softened, about 5 minutes.
6. Add diced carrot and diced celery to the pot and cook for an additional 3-4 minutes.
7. Pour in low-sodium chicken broth and bring to a simmer.
8. Add chopped kale and cooked meatballs to the pot and simmer for 10-15 minutes.
9. Season with salt and pepper to taste.
10. Serve hot, garnished with fresh parsley if desired.

Nutrition Facts (per serving):

- Calories: 250
- Carbs: 15g
- Protein: 25g
- Fat: 10g

22. Grilled Shrimp and Vegetable Spring Rolls with Sesame Soy Dip

Prep.Time: 30 min

Cook Time: 10 min

Serving: 6

Beverage pairing: Green Tea

Ingredients:

- 12 large shrimp, peeled and deveined
- 12 rice paper wrappers
- 1 cup shredded lettuce
- 1 carrot, julienned
- 1 cucumber, julienned
- 1 red bell pepper, julienned
- 1/4 cup fresh mint leaves
- 1/4 cup fresh cilantro leaves
- 1/4 cup unsalted peanuts, chopped (optional)
- 1/4 cup reduced-sodium soy sauce
- 2 tablespoons sesame oil
- 1 clove garlic, minced
- 1 teaspoon grated ginger

Preparation:

1. Preheat grill to medium-high heat.
2. Thread shrimp onto skewers and grill for 2-3 minutes per side, until pink and cooked through.
3. Fill a shallow dish with warm water. Dip one rice paper wrapper into the water for a few seconds until softened.
4. Lay the softened rice paper wrapper flat on a clean surface.
5. Place a few shrimp in the center of the wrapper, followed by shredded lettuce, julienned carrot, julienned cucumber, julienned red bell pepper, fresh mint leaves, fresh cilantro leaves, and chopped peanuts (if using).
6. Fold the bottom of the wrapper over the filling, then fold in the sides, and roll up tightly.
7. Repeat with remaining wrappers and filling ingredients.
8. In a small bowl, whisk together reduced-sodium soy sauce, sesame oil, rice vinegar, honey or low-calorie sweetener, minced garlic, and grated ginger to make the dip.
9. Serve grilled shrimp and vegetable spring rolls with sesame soy dip on the side.

Nutrition Facts (per serving, serving size: 2 spring rolls with dip):

- Calories: 250
- Carbs: 20g
- Protein: 18g
- Fat: 10g

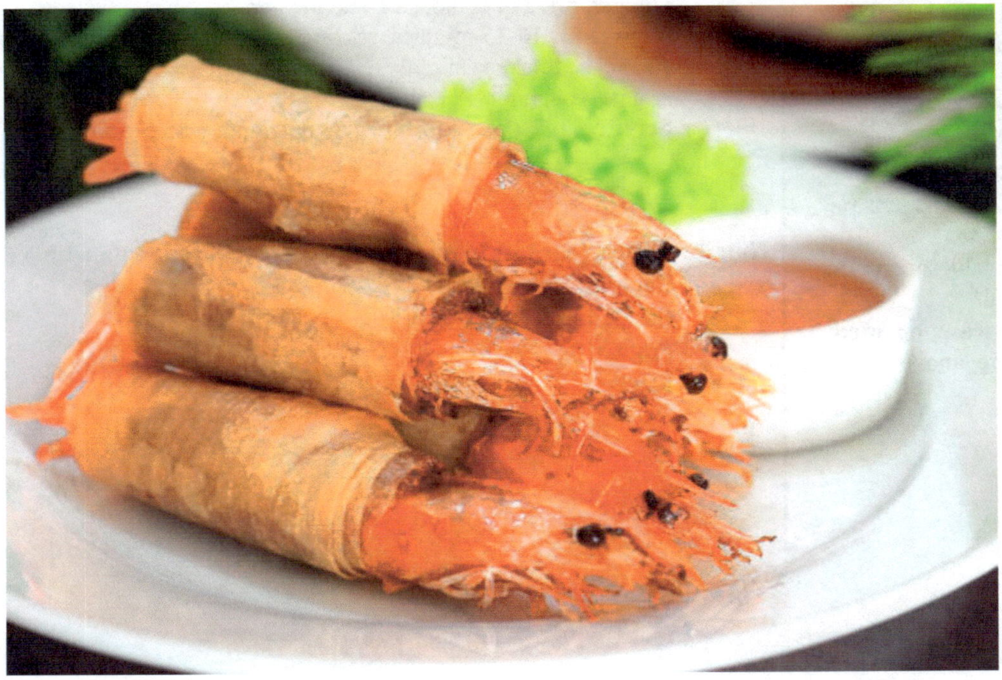

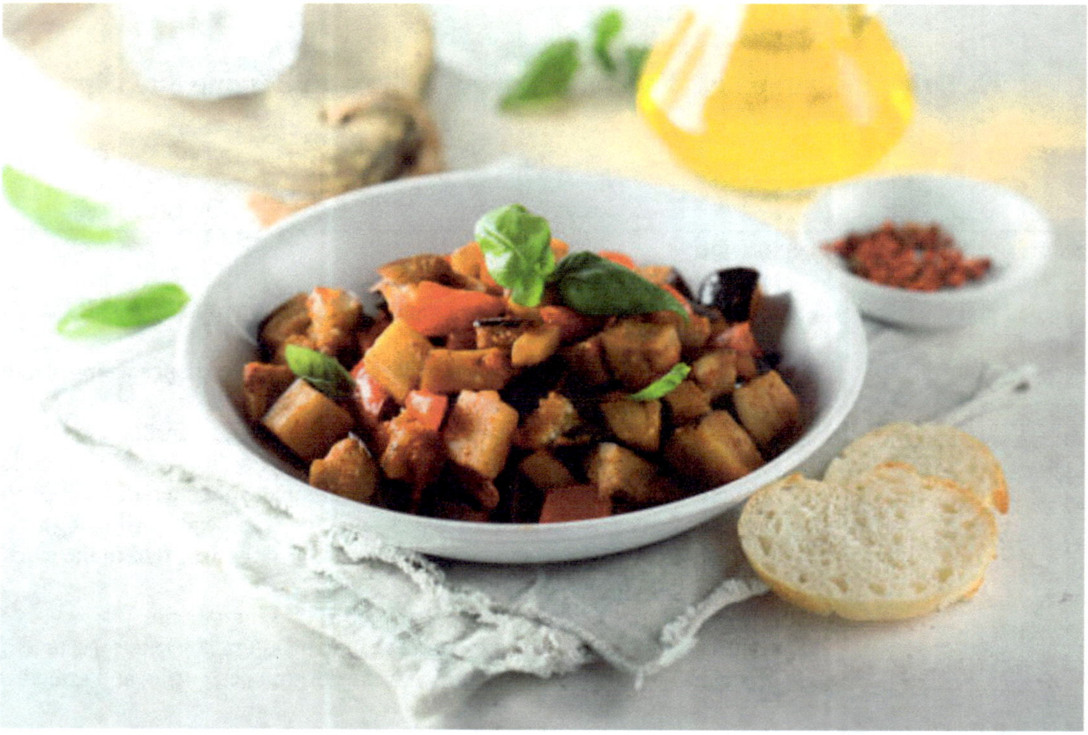

23. Eggplant and Zucchini Caponata with Whole Grain Crackers

Prep.Time: 15 min

Cook Time: 25 min

Serving: 6

Beverage pairing: Herbal Tea

Ingredients:

- 1 eggplant, diced
- 2 zucchinis, diced
- 1 onion, diced
- 2 cloves garlic, minced
- 1 can (14 oz) diced tomatoes
- 1/4 cup chopped green olives
- 2 tablespoons capers
- 2 tablespoons red wine vinegar
- 1 tablespoon olive oil
- 1 teaspoon dried oregano

Preparation:

1. Heat olive oil in a large skillet over medium heat. Add diced onion and minced garlic, and sauté until softened, about 5 minutes.
2. Add diced eggplant and diced zucchini to the skillet, and cook until vegetables are tender, about 8-10 minutes.
3. Stir in diced tomatoes (with juices), chopped green olives, capers, red wine vinegar, dried oregano, salt, and pepper.
4. Simmer for 10-15 minutes, stirring occasionally, until flavors meld together and sauce thickens slightly.
5. Adjust seasoning if necessary.
6. Serve eggplant and zucchini caponata with whole grain crackers on the side.

Nutrition Facts (per serving, serving size: 1/2 cup caponata with 4 crackers):

- Calories: 120
- Carbs: 15g
- Protein: 3g
- Fat: 6g

24. Quinoa and Vegetable Stuffed Poblano Peppers

Prep.Time: 20 min

Cook Time: 30 min

Serving: 4

Beverage pairing: Herbal Tea

Ingredients:

- 4 large poblano peppers
- 1 cup cooked quinoa
- 1 can (15 oz) black beans, drained and rinsed
- 1 cup diced tomatoes
- 1 cup corn kernels (fresh or frozen)
- 1/2 cup diced red onion
- 1/4 cup chopped fresh cilantro
- 1 teaspoon ground cumin
- 1/2 teaspoon chili powder
- Lime wedges for serving

Preparation:

1. Preheat oven to 375°F (190°C).
2. Cut a slit lengthwise along one side of each poblano pepper, leaving the stem intact. Remove seeds and membranes.
3. In a large bowl, combine cooked quinoa, black beans, diced tomatoes, corn kernels, diced red onion, chopped fresh cilantro, ground cumin, chili powder, salt, and pepper.
4. Stuff each poblano pepper with the quinoa and vegetable mixture.
5. Place stuffed poblano peppers in a baking dish.
6. If using, sprinkle shredded reduced-fat cheese over the top of each stuffed pepper.
7. Bake in the preheated oven for 25-30 minutes, or until peppers are tender and filling is heated through.
8. Serve hot with lime wedges on the side.

Nutrition Facts (per serving):

- Calories: 220
- Carbs: 35g
- Protein: 11g
- Fat: 4g

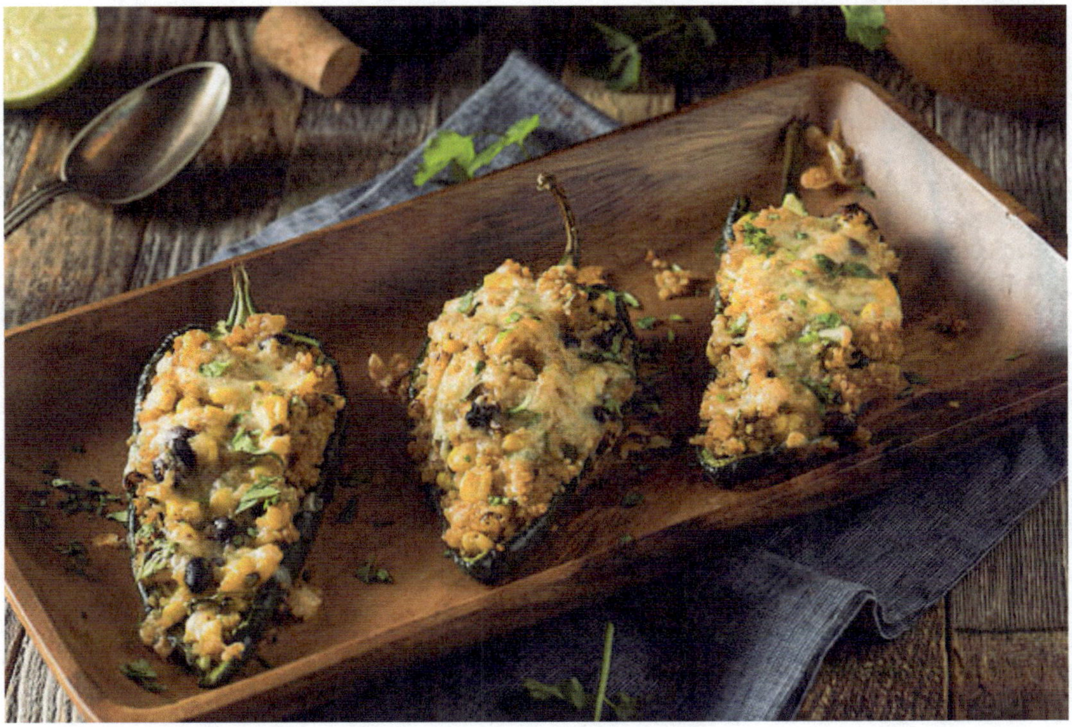

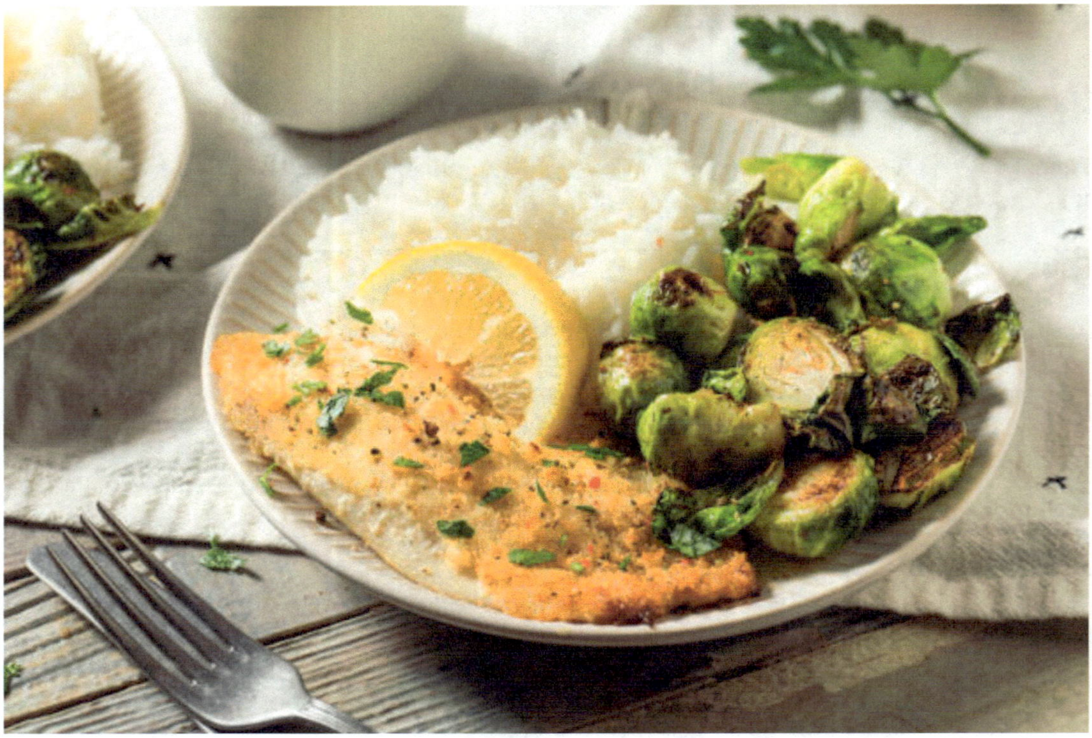

25. Lemon Garlic Tilapia with Roasted Brussels Sprouts

Prep.Time:	Cook Time:	Serving:	Beverage pairing:
10 min	20 min	6	Green Tea

Ingredients:

- 4 tilapia fillets
- 2 tablespoons olive oil
- 2 cloves garlic, minced
- Zest and juice of 1 lemon
- 1 teaspoon dried thyme
- Salt and pepper to taste
- 1 pound Brussels sprouts, trimmed and halved

Preparation:

1. Preheat oven to 400°F (200°C).
2. In a small bowl, whisk together olive oil, minced garlic, lemon zest, lemon juice, dried thyme, salt, and pepper to make the marinade.
3. Place tilapia fillets in a baking dish and pour marinade over them. Turn to coat evenly.
4. Arrange halved Brussels sprouts around the tilapia fillets in the baking dish.
5. Bake in the preheated oven for 15-20 minutes, or until tilapia is cooked through and Brussels sprouts are tender.
6. Serve hot.

Nutrition Facts (per serving):

- Calories: 200
- Carbs: 10g
- Protein: 25g
- Fat: 8g

26. Chicken and Broccoli Quiche with Almond Flour Crust

Prep.Time: 15 min

Cook Time: 40 min

Serving: 6

Beverage pairing: Iced Tea

Ingredients:

- 1 1/2 cups almond flour
- 1/4 teaspoon salt
- 1/4 cup unsalted butter, melted

Quiche Filling:

- 1 cup cooked chicken breast, diced
- 1 cup broccoli florets, chopped
- 4 large eggs
- 1/2 cup unsweetened almond milk
- 1/4 cup grated Parmesan cheese
- 1/4 teaspoon garlic powder
- Salt and pepper to taste

Preparation:

1. Preheat the oven to 350°F (175°C).
2. In a bowl, mix almond flour and salt. Stir in melted butter until well combined.
3. Press the mixture into a greased pie dish to form the crust. Bake for 10 minutes.
4. Meanwhile, in another bowl, whisk together eggs, almond milk, Parmesan cheese, garlic powder, salt, and pepper.
5. Spread diced chicken and chopped broccoli evenly over the pre-baked crust.
6. Pour the egg mixture over the chicken and broccoli.
7. Bake for 25-30 minutes, or until the quiche is set and the top is golden brown.
8. Let it cool for a few minutes before slicing. Garnish with chopped parsley if desired.

Nutrition Facts (per serving):

- Calories: 220
- Carbs: 35g
- Protein: 11g
- Fat: 4g

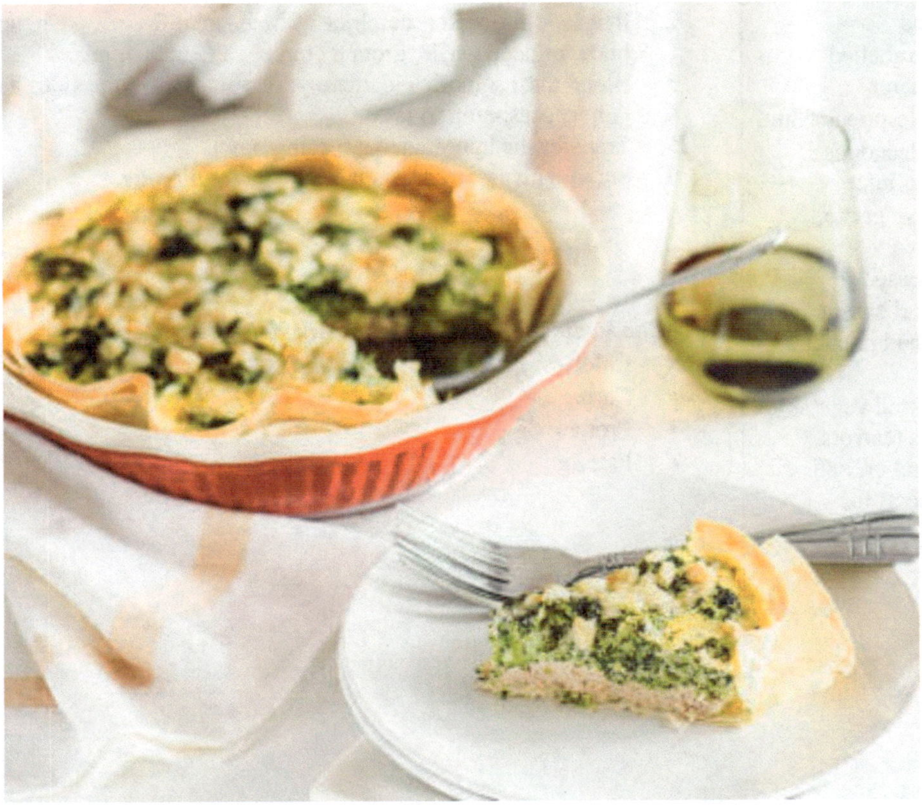

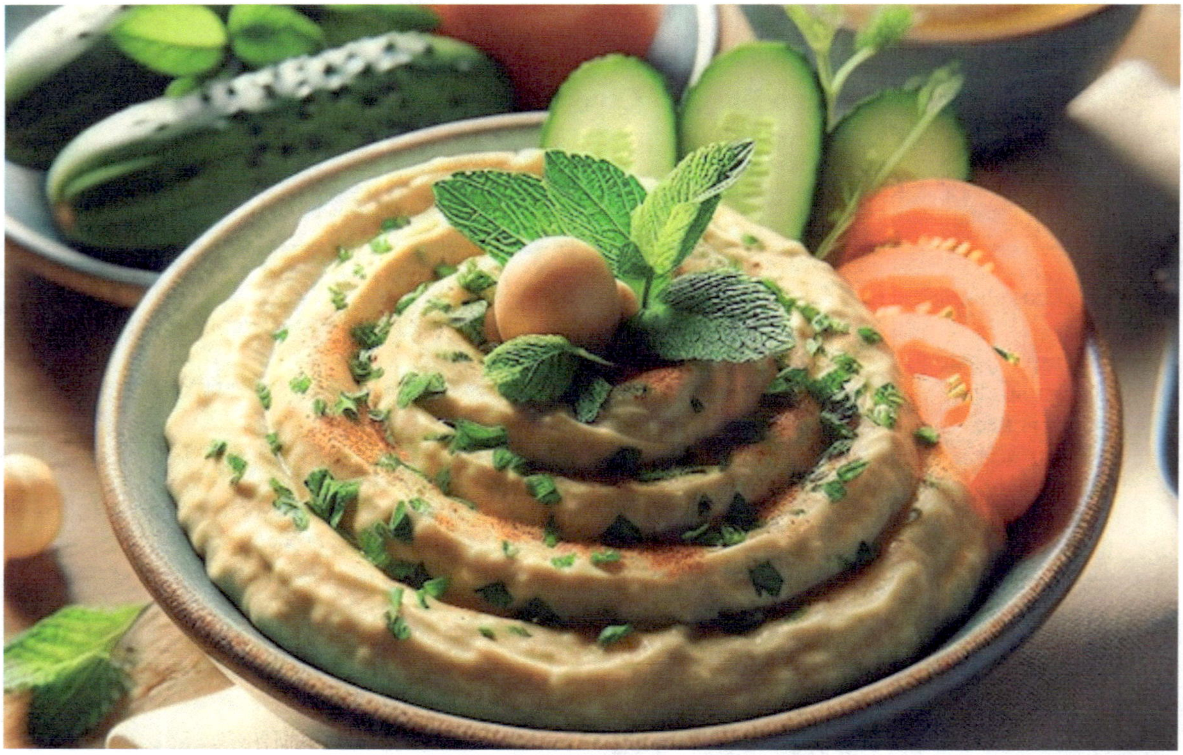

27. Cauliflower and Edamame Hummus with Veggie Sticks

Prep.Time: 10 min

Cook Time: 10 min

Serving: 6

Beverage pairing: Herbal Tea

Ingredients:

- 2 cups cauliflower florets
- 1 cup shelled edamame
- 2 tablespoons tahini
- 2 tablespoons lemon juice
- 1 clove garlic, minced
- 1/4 teaspoon ground cumin
- Salt and pepper to taste
- Assorted vegetable sticks (carrots, cucumber, bell peppers) for serving

Preparation:

1. Steam cauliflower florets and edamame until tender.
2. In a food processor, combine steamed cauliflower, edamame, tahini, lemon juice, minced garlic, ground cumin, salt, and pepper.
3. Blend until smooth and creamy, scraping down the sides as needed.
4. Adjust seasoning to taste.
5. Transfer the hummus to a serving bowl.
6. Serve with assorted vegetable sticks for dipping.

Nutrition Facts (per serving, without vegetable sticks):

- Calories: 120
- Carbs: 7g
- Protein: 6g
- Fat: 8g

28. Turkey and Spinach Stuffed Acorn Squash

Prep.Time: 15 min

Cook Time: 40 min

Serving: 4

Beverage pairing: HerbalTea

Ingredients:

- 2 acorn squashes, halved and seeded
- 1 tablespoon olive oil
- 1 small onion, diced
- 1 clove garlic, minced
- 1 pound ground turkey
- 2 cups fresh spinach, chopped
- 1/4 cup grated Parmesan cheese
- Salt and pepper to taste
- Chopped fresh parsley for garnish (optional)

Preparation:

1. Preheat oven to 400°F (200°C).
2. Place acorn squash halves on a baking sheet, cut side up. Brush the cut sides with olive oil and sprinkle with salt and pepper.
3. Bake squash in the preheated oven for 30-35 minutes, or until tender.
4. Meanwhile, heat olive oil in a skillet over medium heat. Add diced onion and minced garlic, and sauté until softened.
5. Add ground turkey to the skillet and cook until browned, breaking it into small pieces as it cooks.
6. Stir in chopped spinach and cook until wilted.
7. Remove skillet from heat and stir in grated Parmesan cheese. Season with salt and pepper to taste.
8. Fill each roasted acorn squash half with the turkey and spinach mixture.
9. Garnish with chopped fresh parsley, if desired, before serving.

Nutrition Facts (per serving):

- Calories: 280
- Carbs: 20g
- Protein: 25g
- Fat: 12g

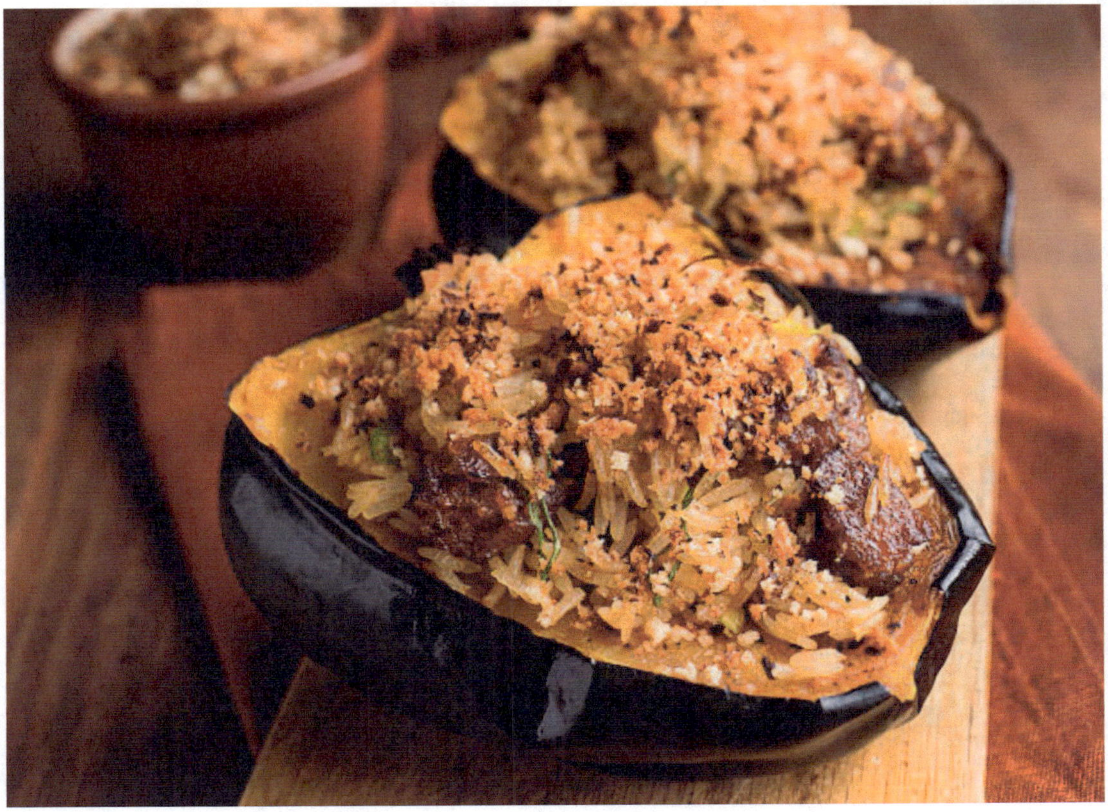

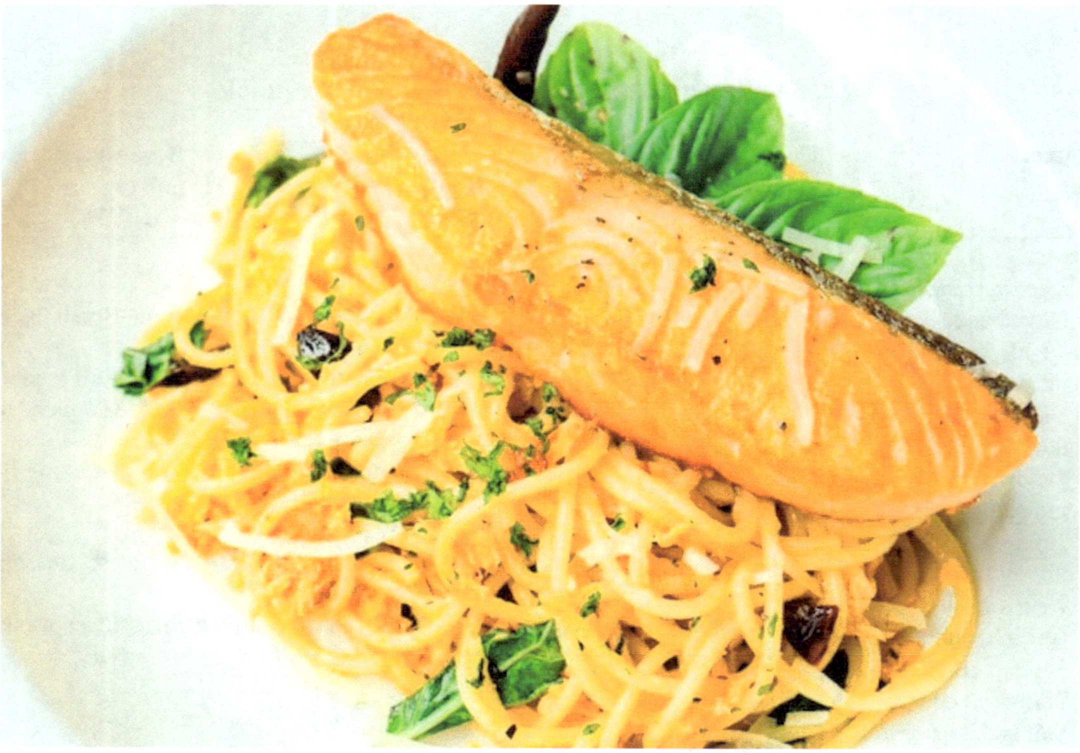

29. Baked Salmon with Dill and Lemon Zucchini Noodles

Prep.Time: 15 min

Cook Time: 15 min

Serving: 4

Beverage pairing: Herbal Tea

Ingredients:

- 4 salmon fillets
- 2 tablespoons olive oil
- 2 tablespoons chopped fresh dill
- Zest and juice of 1 lemon
- Salt and pepper to taste
- 4 medium zucchinis, spiralized into noodles
- 2 cloves garlic, minced

Preparation:

1. Preheat oven to 400°F (200°C).
2. Place salmon fillets on a baking sheet lined with parchment paper.
3. In a small bowl, mix together olive oil, chopped fresh dill, lemon zest, lemon juice, salt, and pepper.
4. Brush the dill and lemon mixture over the salmon fillets.
5. Bake in the preheated oven for 12-15 minutes, or until salmon is cooked through and flakes easily with a fork.
6. Meanwhile, heat olive oil in a large skillet over medium heat. Add minced garlic and cook until fragrant.
7. Add zucchini noodles to the skillet and sauté for 3-4 minutes, or until tender.
8. Season zucchini noodles with salt and pepper to taste.
9. Serve baked salmon fillets over lemon garlic zucchini noodles.

Nutrition Facts (per serving):

- Calories: 300
- Carbs: 10g
- Protein: 30g
- Fat: 15g

30. Zucchini and Tomato Gratin with Mozzarella

Prep.Time: 15 min

Cook Time: 35- 40 min

Serving: 4

Beverage pairing: HerbalTea

Ingredients:

- 4 medium zucchinis, thinly sliced
- 2 large tomatoes, thinly sliced
- 2 cloves garlic, minced
- 1/4 cup grated Parmesan cheese
- 1/2 cup shredded mozzarella cheese
- 2 tablespoons olive oil
- 1 teaspoon dried oregano
- Salt and pepper to taste

Preparation:

1. Preheat oven to 375°F (190°C).
2. In a large bowl, toss together thinly sliced zucchinis and minced garlic with olive oil, dried oregano, salt, and pepper.
3. Arrange half of the zucchini slices in a greased baking dish, overlapping slightly.
4. Layer half of the tomato slices on top of the zucchini slices.
5. Sprinkle grated Parmesan cheese over the tomatoes.
6. Repeat the layers with the remaining zucchini slices and tomato slices.
7. Top with shredded mozzarella cheese.
8. Cover the baking dish with aluminum foil and bake in the preheated oven for 20 minutes.
9. Remove the foil and bake for an additional 15-20 minutes, or until the vegetables are tender and the cheese is golden brown.
10. Garnish with chopped fresh basil, if desired, before serving.

Nutrition Facts (per serving):

- Calories: 180
- Carbs: 8g
- Protein: 8g
- Fat: 12g

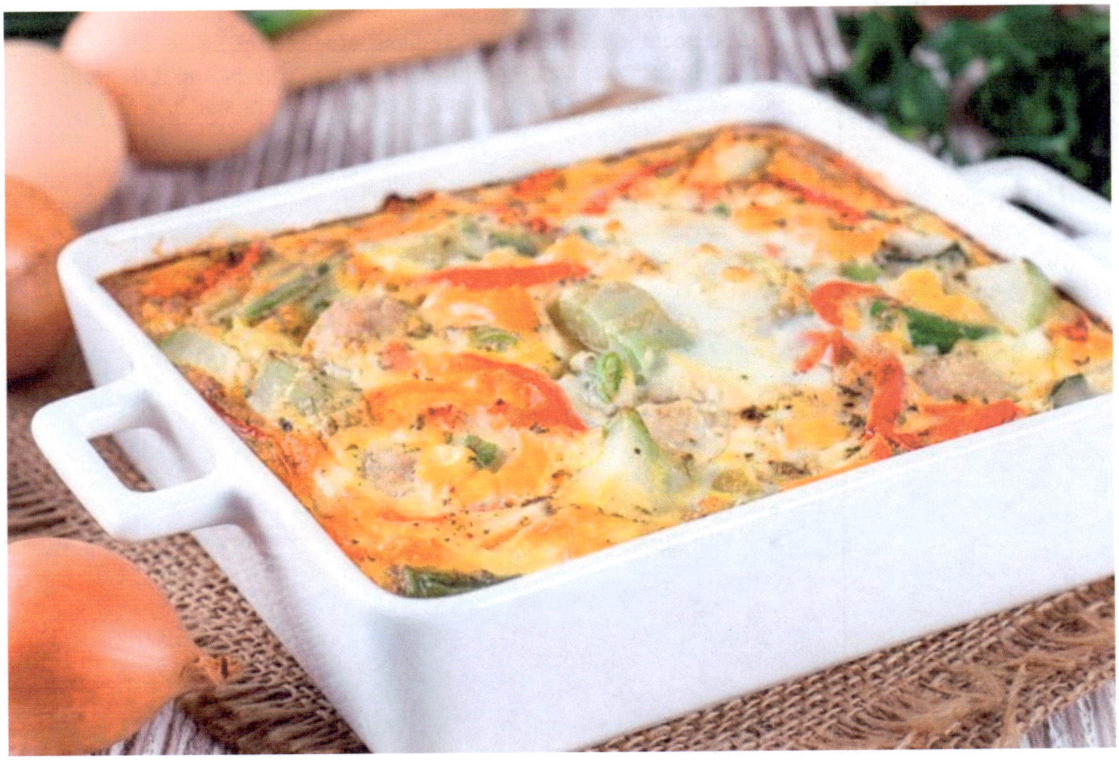

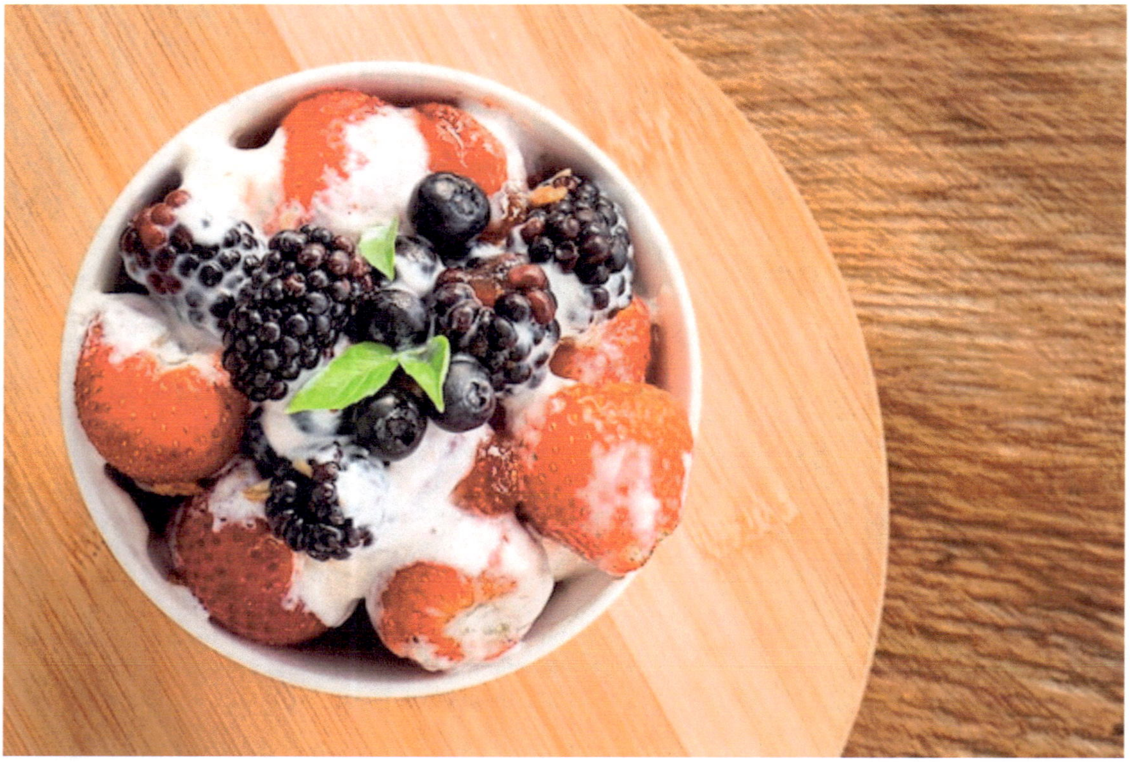

31. Greek Yogurt Parfait with Berries and Almond Granola

Prep.Time:	Cook Time:	Serving:	Beverage pairing:
5 min	0 min	1	Black Coffee

Ingredients:

- 1 cup Greek yogurt (unsweetened)
- 1/2 cup mixed berries (such as strawberries, blueberries, raspberries)
- 1/4 cup almond granola (unsweetened)
- 1 tablespoon honey or low-calorie sweetener (optional)

Preparation:

1. In a serving glass or bowl, layer Greek yogurt, mixed berries, and almond granola.
2. Repeat the layers until ingredients are used up.
3. Drizzle honey or low-calorie sweetener over the top if desired.
4. Serve immediately as a nutritious breakfast or snack.

Nutrition Facts (per serving):

- Calories: 250
- Carbs: 25g
- Protein: 20g
- Fat: 8g

32. Shrimp and Avocado Cilantro Lime Bowl

Prep.Time: 15 min

Cook Time: 10 min

Serving: 2

Beverage pairing: Herbal Tea

Ingredients:

- 8 oz shrimp, peeled and deveined
- 1 tablespoon olive oil
- 1/4 teaspoon chili powder
- Salt and pepper to taste
- 2 cups cooked quinoa
- 1 avocado, sliced
- 1/4 cup chopped fresh cilantro
- Juice of 1 lime
- Lime wedges for serving

Preparation:

1. In a bowl, toss shrimp with olive oil, chili powder, salt, and pepper until well coated.
2. Heat a skillet over medium-high heat. Add shrimp and cook for 2-3 minutes per side, or until pink and cooked through.
3. Divide cooked quinoa between serving bowls.
4. Top with cooked shrimp, sliced avocado, and chopped fresh cilantro.
5. Drizzle lime juice over the top.
6. Serve with lime wedges on the side.

Nutrition Facts (per serving):

- Calories: 400
- Carbs: 30g
- Protein: 25g
- Fat: 20g

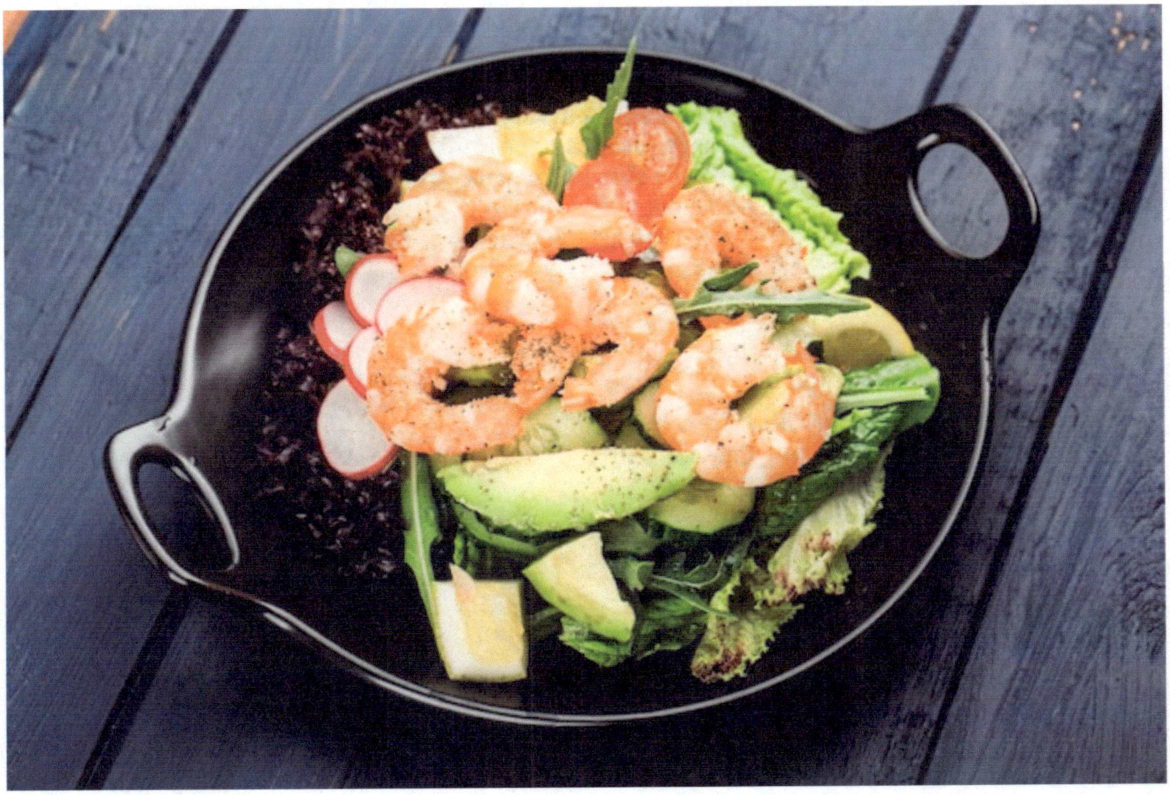

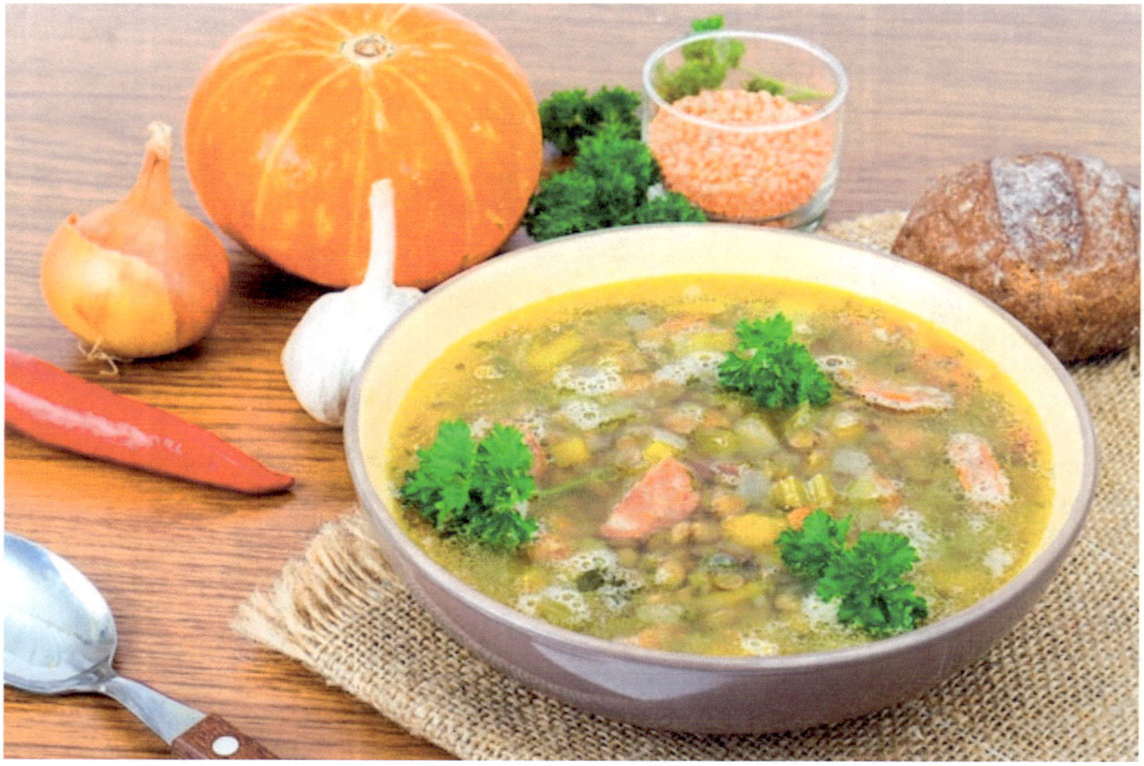

33. Turkey and Cabbage Roll Soup

Prep.Time:	Cook Time:	Serving:	Beverage pairing:
15 min	25 min	6	Iced Tea

Ingredients:

- 1 tablespoon olive oil
- 1 onion, diced
- 2 cloves garlic, minced
- 1 pound ground turkey
- 4 cups low-sodium chicken broth
- 1 can (14 oz) diced tomatoes
- 2 cups shredded cabbage
- 1 carrot, diced
- 1 celery stalk, diced
- 1/4 cup chopped fresh parsley
- Salt and pepper to taste

Preparation:

1. Heat olive oil in a large pot over medium heat. Add diced onion and minced garlic, and sauté until softened.
2. Add ground turkey to the pot and cook until browned, breaking it into small pieces as it cooks.
3. Stir in low-sodium chicken broth, diced tomatoes (with juices), shredded cabbage, diced carrot, and diced celery.
4. Bring the soup to a simmer and cook for 20-25 minutes, or until vegetables are tender.
5. Stir in chopped fresh parsley and season with salt and pepper to taste.
6. Serve hot.

Nutrition Facts (per serving):

- Calories: 250
- Carbs: 10g
- Protein: 20g
- Fat: 15g

34. Eggplant and Chickpea Lettuce Wraps with Mint Yogurt Sauce

Prep.Time: 15 min | **Cook Time:** 25 min | **Serving:** 4 | **Beverage pairing:** Green Tea

Ingredients:

- 1 large eggplant, diced
- 1 can (15 oz) chickpeas, drained and rinsed
- 2 tablespoons olive oil
- 1 teaspoon ground cumin
- 1 teaspoon paprika
- Salt and pepper to taste
- 1/2 cup Greek yogurt (unsweetened)
- 2 tablespoons chopped fresh mint
- 1 tablespoon lemon juice
- 8 large lettuce leaves (such as romaine or butter lettuce)

Preparation:

1. Preheat oven to 400°F (200°C).
2. In a bowl, toss diced eggplant and drained chickpeas with olive oil, ground cumin, paprika, salt, and pepper until well coated.
3. Spread the seasoned eggplant and chickpeas out on a baking sheet lined with parchment paper.
4. Roast in the preheated oven for 20-25 minutes, or until eggplant is tender and chickpeas are crispy.
5. In a small bowl, mix together Greek yogurt, chopped fresh mint, and lemon juice to make the sauce.
6. To assemble the lettuce wraps, place a spoonful of roasted eggplant and chickpeas on each lettuce leaf.
7. Drizzle mint yogurt sauce over the top.
8. Serve immediately.

Nutrition Facts (per serving, serving size: 2 lettuce wraps):

- Calories: 200
- Carbs: 20g
- Protein: 10g
- Fat: 10g

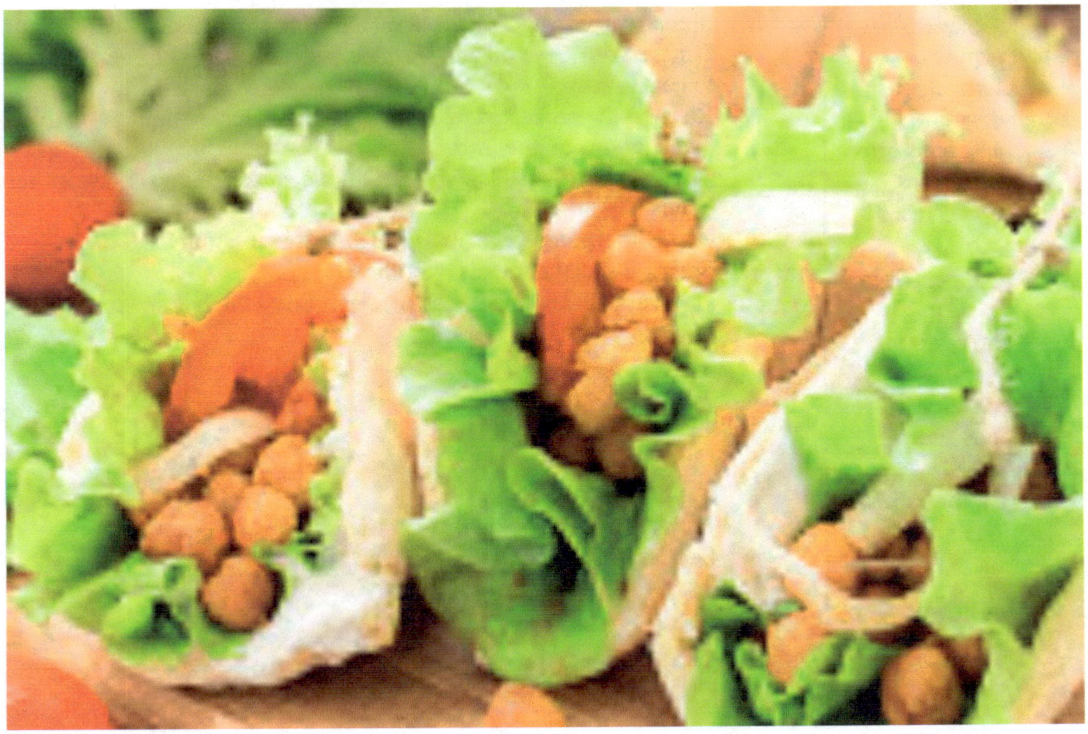

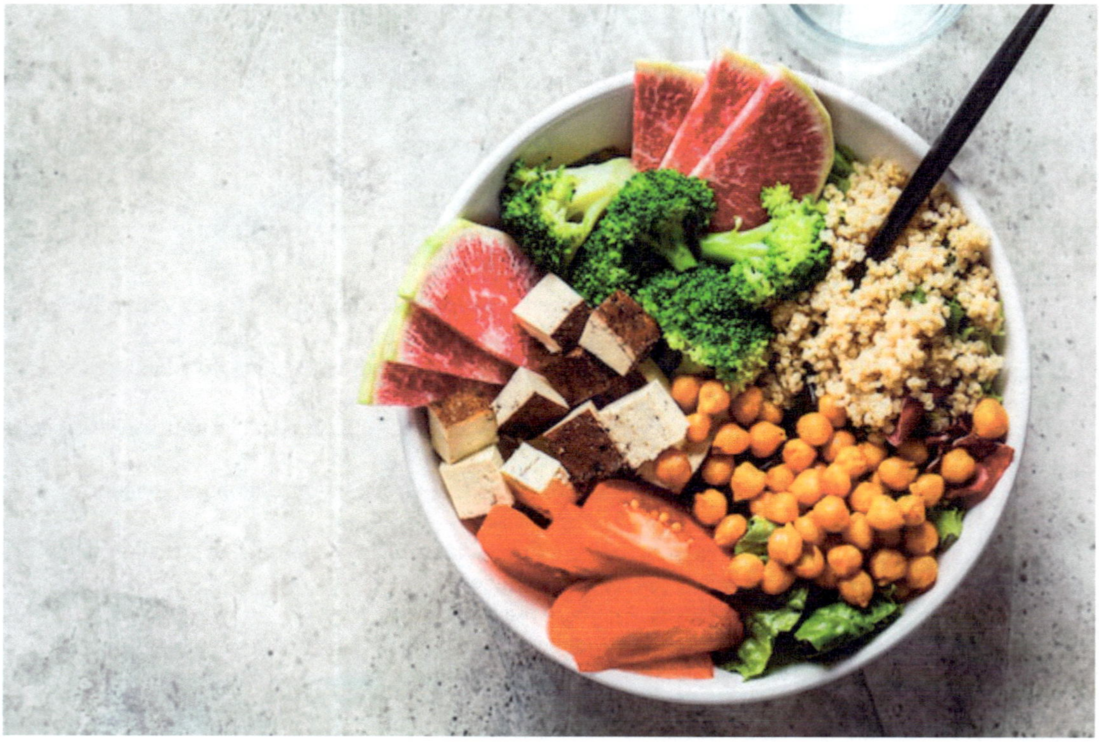

35. Quinoa and Roasted Vegetable Buddha Bowl

Prep.Time: 15 min

Cook Time: 25 min

Serving: 4

Beverage pairing: Iced Tea

Ingredients:

- 1 cup quinoa
- 2 cups mixed vegetables (such as bell peppers, zucchini, cherry tomatoes)
- 2 tablespoons olive oil
- 1 teaspoon dried oregano
- Salt and pepper to taste
- 1/4 cup hummus (unsweetened)
- 1/4 cup sliced almonds
- Chopped fresh parsley for garnish (optional)

Preparation:

1. Preheat oven to 400°F (200°C).
2. Cook quinoa according to package instructions.
3. Spread mixed vegetables out on a baking sheet lined with parchment paper.
4. Drizzle with olive oil and sprinkle with dried oregano, salt, and pepper. Toss to coat evenly.
5. Roast in the preheated oven for 20-25 minutes, or until vegetables are tender and slightly caramelized.
6. To assemble the Buddha bowls, divide cooked quinoa between serving bowls.
7. Top with roasted vegetables and a dollop of hummus.
8. Sprinkle sliced almonds over the top.
9. Garnish with chopped fresh parsley, if desired, before serving.

Nutrition Facts (per serving):

- Calories: 300
- Carbs: 30g
- Protein: 10g
- Fat: 15g

36. Cumin-Spiced Cauliflower and Chickpea Tacos

Prep.Time: 15 min | **Cook Time:** 25 min | **Serving:** 4 | **Beverage pairing:** Herbal Tea

Ingredients:

- 1 head cauliflower, cut into florets
- 1 can (15 oz) chickpeas, drained and rinsed
- 2 tablespoons olive oil
- 1 tablespoon ground cumin
- 1 teaspoon paprika
- 1/2 teaspoon garlic powder
- Salt and pepper to taste
- 8 small whole wheat or corn tortillas
- Toppings: diced tomatoes, shredded lettuce, sliced avocado, Greek yogurt (unsweetened), lime wedges

Preparation:

1. Preheat oven to 400°F (200°C).
2. In a bowl, toss cauliflower florets and drained chickpeas with olive oil, ground cumin, paprika, garlic powder, salt, and pepper until well coated.
3. Spread the seasoned cauliflower and chickpeas out on a baking sheet lined with parchment paper.
4. Roast in the preheated oven for 20-25 minutes, or until cauliflower is tender and chickpeas are crispy.
5. Warm tortillas according to package instructions.
6. To assemble the tacos, fill each tortilla with roasted cauliflower and chickpeas.
7. Top with diced tomatoes, shredded lettuce, sliced avocado, and a dollop of Greek yogurt.
8. Serve with lime wedges on the side for squeezing.

Nutrition Facts (per serving, serving size: 2 tacos):

- Calories: 300
- Carbs: 35g
- Protein: 10g
- Fat: 14g

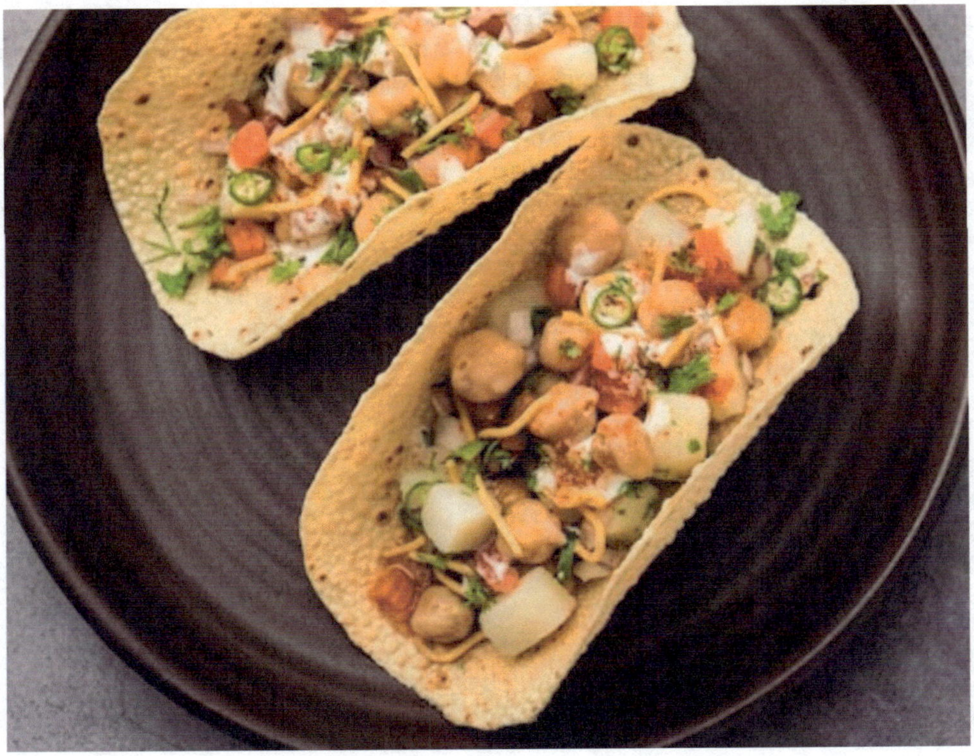

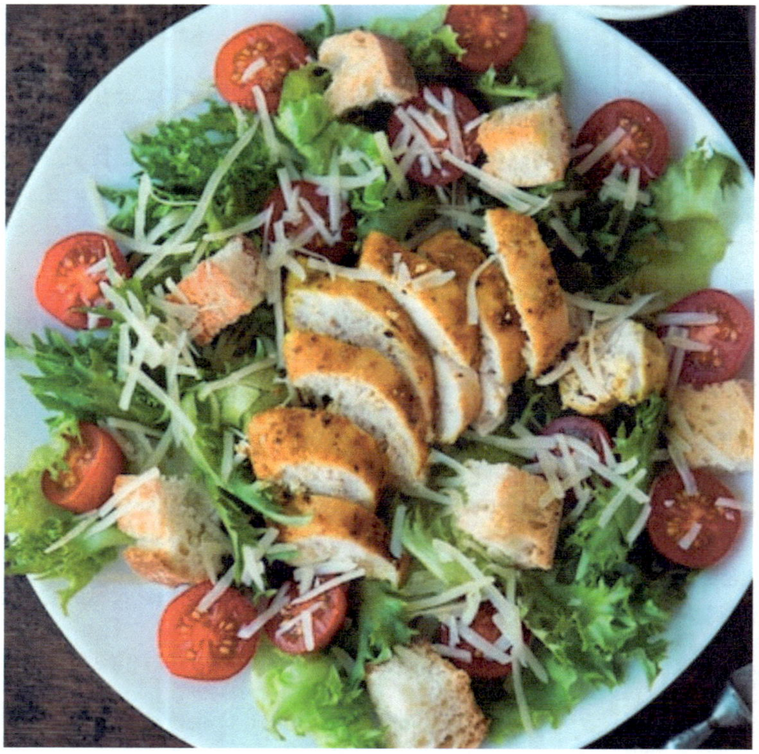

37. Grilled Chicken and Asparagus Salad with Mustard Vinaigrette

Prep.Time: 15 min

Cook Time: 15 min

Serving: 4

Beverage pairing: Herbal Tea

Ingredients:

- 4 boneless, skinless chicken breasts
- 1 bunch asparagus, trimmed
- 2 tablespoons olive oil
- Salt and pepper to taste
- 6 cups mixed salad greens
- 1/4 cup sliced almonds
- 1/4 cup crumbled feta cheese
- 2 tablespoons olive oil
- 1 tablespoon balsamic vinegar
- 1 teaspoon Dijon mustard

Preparation:

1. Preheat grill to medium-high heat.
2. Brush chicken breasts and trimmed asparagus with olive oil, and season with salt and pepper.
3. Grill chicken for 6-8 minutes per side, or until cooked through, and grill asparagus for 3-4 minutes per side, or until tender.
4. Let chicken rest for a few minutes before slicing.
5. In a small bowl, whisk together olive oil, balsamic vinegar, Dijon mustard, salt, and pepper to make the vinaigrette.
6. In a large bowl, toss mixed salad greens with sliced almonds and crumbled feta cheese.
7. Divide salad greens between serving plates.
8. Top with sliced grilled chicken and grilled asparagus.
9. Drizzle mustard vinaigrette over the top.
10. Serve immediately.

Nutrition Facts (per serving):

- Calories: 350
- Carbs: 8g
- Protein: 30g
- Fat: 22g

38. Stuffed Portobello Mushrooms with Turkey and Spinach

Prep.Time: 15 min

Cook Time: 25 min

Serving: 4

Beverage pairing: Iced Tea

Ingredients:

- 4 large portobello mushrooms, stems removed
- 1 tablespoon olive oil
- 1 small onion, diced
- 2 cloves garlic, minced
- 1 pound ground turkey
- 2 cups fresh spinach, chopped
- 1/4 cup grated Parmesan cheese
- Salt and pepper to taste
- Chopped fresh parsley for garnish (optional)

Preparation:

1. Preheat oven to 375°F (190°C).
2. Place portobello mushrooms on a baking sheet lined with parchment paper.
3. In a skillet, heat olive oil over medium heat. Add diced onion and minced garlic, and sauté until softened.
4. Add ground turkey to the skillet and cook until browned, breaking it into small pieces as it cooks.
5. Stir in chopped fresh spinach and cook until wilted.
6. Remove skillet from heat and stir in grated Parmesan cheese. Season with salt and pepper to taste.
7. Spoon turkey and spinach mixture into the cavity of each portobello mushroom.
8. Bake in the preheated oven for 20-25 minutes, or until mushrooms are tender and filling is heated through.
9. Garnish with chopped fresh parsley, if desired, before serving.

Nutrition Facts (per serving):

- Calories: 250
- Carbs: 7g
- Protein: 30g
- Fat: 12g

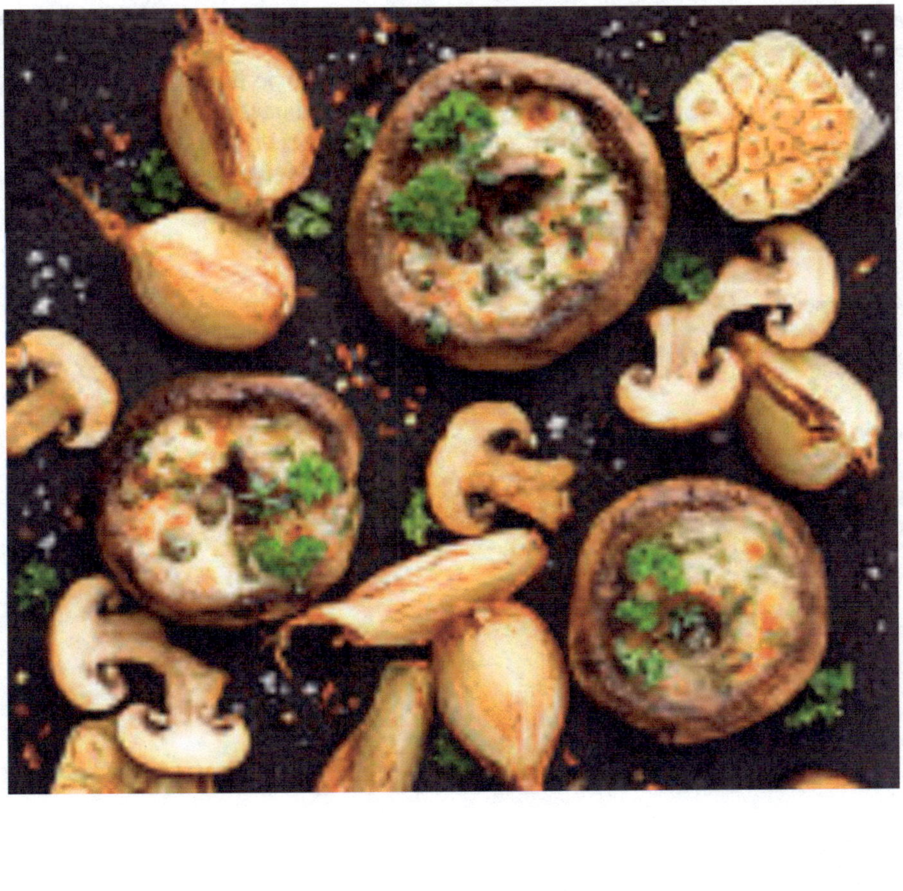

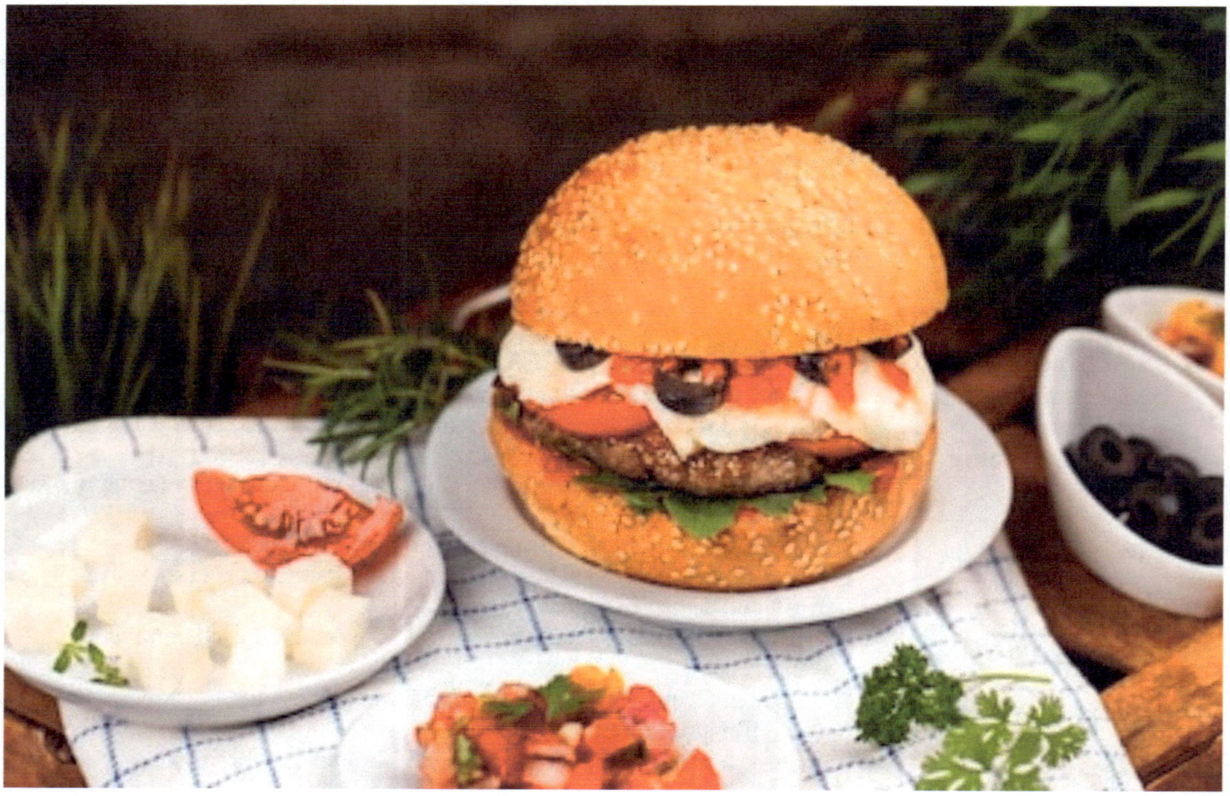

39. Roasted Red Pepper and Feta Turkey Burger with Bun

Prep.Time: 10 min

Cook Time: 15 min

Serving: 4

Beverage pairing: Herbal Tea

Ingredients:

- 1 pound ground turkey
- 1/4 cup chopped roasted red peppers
- 1/4 cup crumbled feta cheese
- 1 tablespoon chopped fresh parsley
- 1 teaspoon garlic powder
- Salt and pepper to taste
- 4 large lettuce leaves
- Toppings: sliced tomato, sliced red onion, sliced avocado (optional)

Preparation:

1. Preheat grill to medium-high heat.
2. In a bowl, mix together ground turkey, chopped roasted red peppers, crumbled feta cheese, chopped fresh parsley, garlic powder, salt, and pepper until well combined.
3. Divide the mixture into 4 equal portions and shape into burger patties.
4. Grill turkey burgers for 6-8 minutes per side, or until cooked through.
5. Place each grilled turkey burger on a large lettuce leaf.
6. Top with sliced tomato, sliced red onion, and sliced avocado if desired.
7. Wrap lettuce leaves around the burgers to form a bun.
8. Serve immediately.

Nutrition Facts (per serving):

- Calories: 280
- Carbs: 5g
- Protein: 25g
- Fat: 18g

40. Lentil and Vegetable Stew with Turmeric

Prep.Time: 10 min

Cook Time: 40 min

Serving: 6

Beverage pairing: Herbal Tea

Ingredients:

- 1 cup dried green lentils, rinsed and drained
- 4 cups low-sodium vegetable broth
- 1 onion, diced
- 2 carrots, diced
- 2 celery stalks, diced
- 2 cloves garlic, minced
- 1 can (14 oz) diced tomatoes
- 1 teaspoon ground turmeric
- 1 teaspoon ground cumin
- Salt and pepper to taste

Preparation:

1. In a large pot, combine dried green lentils, low-sodium vegetable broth, diced onion, diced carrots, diced celery, minced garlic, diced tomatoes (with juices), ground turmeric, and ground cumin.
2. Bring the mixture to a boil over high heat.
3. Reduce heat to low, cover, and simmer for 30-40 minutes, or until lentils and vegetables are tender.
4. Season with salt and pepper to taste.
5. Ladle stew into serving bowls and garnish with chopped fresh parsley if desired.
6. Serve hot.

Nutrition Facts (per serving):

- Calories: 250
- Carbs: 40g
- Protein: 15g
- Fat: 2g

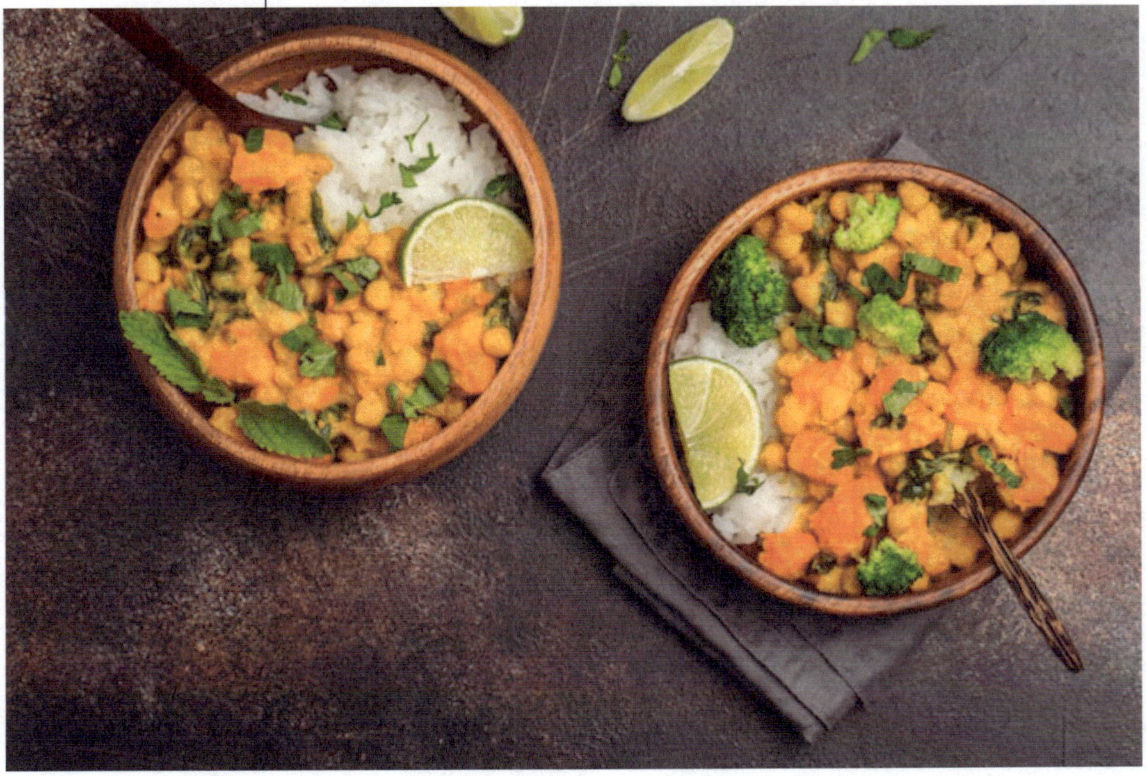

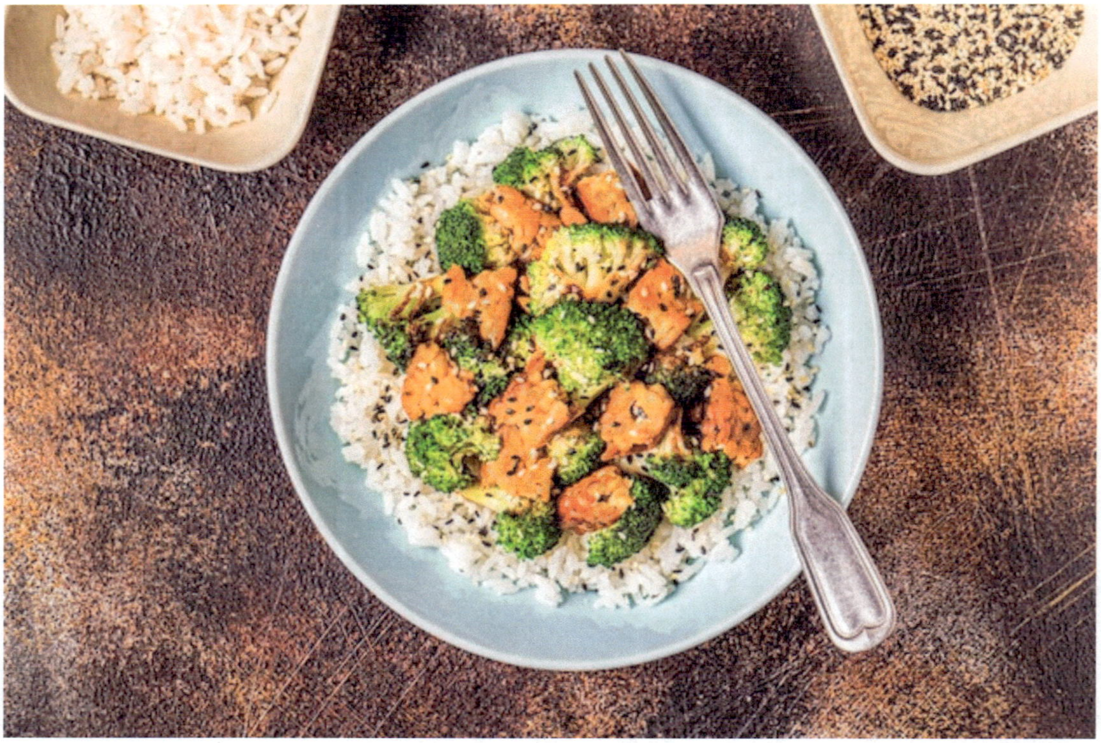

41. Cauliflower and Broccoli Rice Stir-Fry with Tofu

Prep.Time: 15 min

Cook Time: 15 min

Serving: 4

Beverage pairing: Green Tea

Ingredients:

- 1 small head cauliflower
- 1 small head broccoli
- 1 block firm tofu, pressed and cubed
- 2 tablespoons low-sodium soy sauce
- 1 tablespoon sesame oil
- 2 cloves garlic, minced
- 1 teaspoon grated ginger
- 1 carrot, julienned
- 1 bell pepper, thinly sliced
- 2 green onions, sliced
- Salt and pepper to taste

Preparation:

1. Cut cauliflower and broccoli into florets. Working in batches, pulse in a food processor until they resemble rice.
2. In a large skillet or wok, heat sesame oil over medium heat. Add minced garlic and grated ginger, and cook until fragrant.
3. Add cubed tofu to the skillet and cook until lightly browned on all sides.
4. Stir in julienned carrot, sliced bell pepper, and sliced green onions. Cook for 3-4 minutes until vegetables are tender-crisp.
5. Add cauliflower and broccoli rice to the skillet, and drizzle with low-sodium soy sauce. Stir well to combine.
6. Cook for another 3-4 minutes, stirring occasionally, until the "rice" is heated through.
7. Season with salt and pepper to taste.
8. Garnish with sesame seeds if desired before serving.

Nutrition Facts (per serving):

- Calories: 200
- Carbs: 15g
- Protein: 15g
- Fat: 10g

42. Shrimp and Avocado Cucumber with Lime Dressing

Prep.Time: 15 min

Cook Time: 0 min

Serving: 4

Beverage pairing: Herbal Tea

Ingredients:

- 1 pound cooked shrimp, peeled and deveined
- 2 ripe avocados, diced
- 2 cucumbers, halved and seeds removed
- 1/4 cup chopped fresh cilantro
- Juice of 2 limes
- 2 tablespoons olive oil
- 1 teaspoon honey or low-calorie sweetener (optional)
- Salt and pepper to taste

Preparation:

1. In a bowl, combine cooked shrimp, diced avocados, and chopped fresh cilantro.
2. In a separate small bowl, whisk together lime juice, olive oil, honey or low-calorie sweetener (if using), salt, and pepper to make the dressing.
3. Pour the dressing over the shrimp and avocado mixture, and toss gently to coat.
4. Fill each cucumber half with the shrimp and avocado mixture.
5. Serve immediately.

Nutrition Facts (per serving, serving size: 2 cucumber boats):

- Calories: 250
- Carbs: 10g
- Protein: 20g
- Fat: 15g

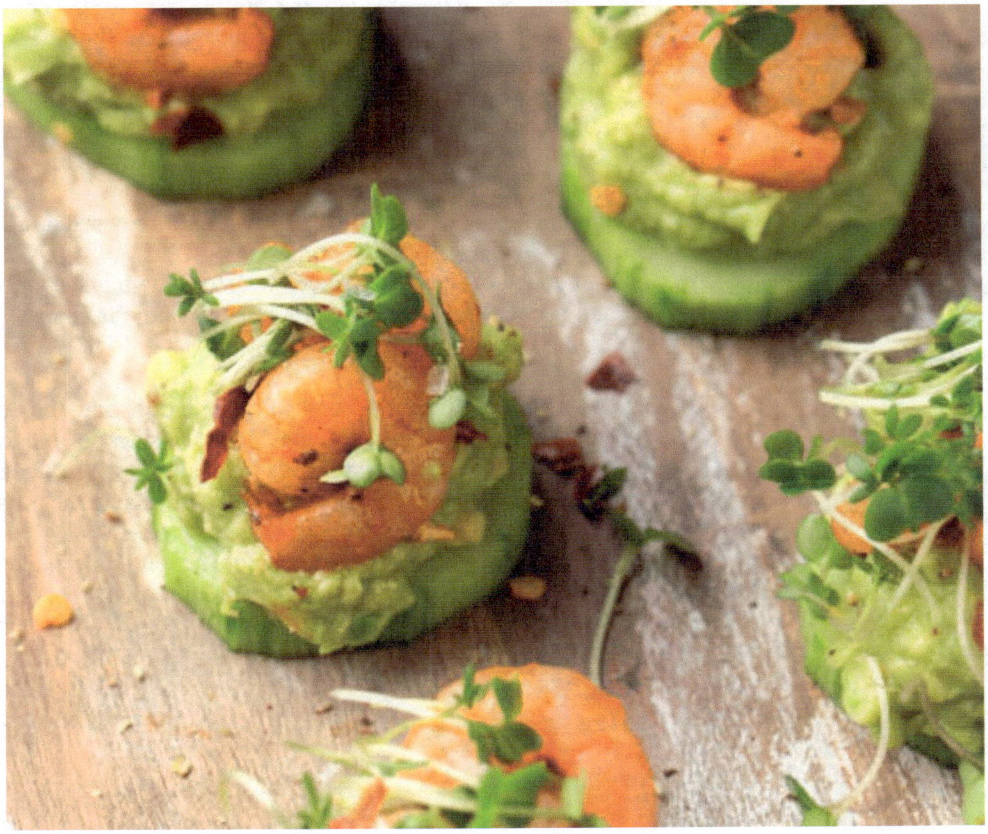

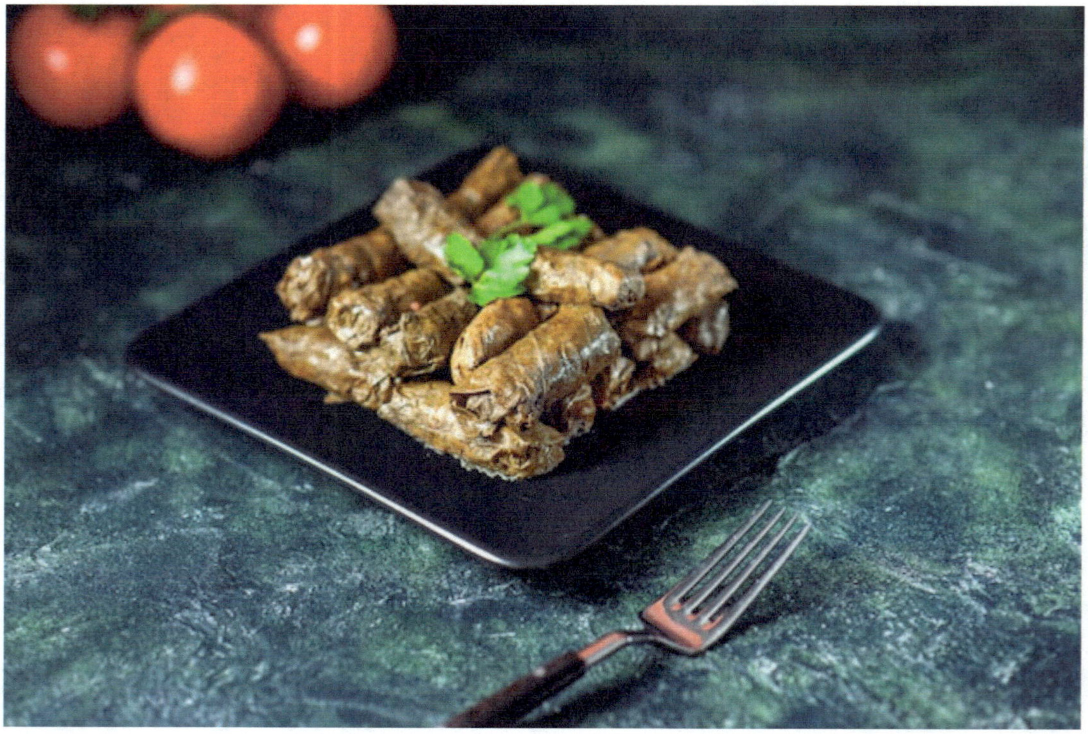

43. Turkey and Spinach Stuffed Cabbage Leaves

Prep.Time: 30 min

Cook Time: 35 min

Serving: 4

Beverage pairing: Iced Tea

Ingredients:

- 1 large head cabbage
- 1 tablespoon olive oil
- 1 small onion, diced
- 2 cloves garlic, minced
- 1 pound ground turkey
- 2 cups chopped fresh spinach
- 1 can (14 oz) diced tomatoes
- 1 teaspoon dried oregano
- Salt and pepper to taste

Preparation:

1. Bring a large pot of water to a boil. Carefully remove the core from the cabbage and place the whole head of cabbage in the boiling water. Cook for 5 minutes, or until the outer leaves are softened. Remove from water and let cool slightly.
2. Gently peel off 8-10 large leaves from the cabbage and set aside.
3. In a skillet, heat olive oil over medium heat. Add diced onion and minced garlic, and sauté until softened.
4. Add ground turkey to the skillet and cook until browned, breaking it into small pieces as it cooks.
5. Stir in chopped fresh spinach, diced tomatoes (with juices), dried oregano, salt, and pepper. Cook for another 5 minutes until the spinach is wilted and the mixture is heated through.
6. Preheat oven to 375°F (190°C).
7. Place a spoonful of the turkey and spinach mixture onto the center of each cabbage leaf. Roll up the leaves, tucking in the sides as you go, to form cabbage rolls. Place the cabbage rolls seam side down in a baking dish.
8. Cover the baking dish with aluminum foil and bake in the preheated oven for 25-30 minutes, or until the cabbage rolls are tender.
9. Garnish with chopped fresh parsley before serving if desired.

Nutrition Facts (per serving, serving size: 2 cabbage rolls):

- Calories: 300
- Carbs: 15g
- Protein: 25g
- Fat: 15g

44. Cauliflower and Chickpea Mash with Garlic and Rosemary

Prep.Time: 15 min

Cook Time: 15 min

Serving: 4

Beverage pairing: Herbal Tea

Ingredients:

- 1 head cauliflower, cut into florets
- 1 can (15 oz) chickpeas, drained and rinsed
- 2 tablespoons olive oil
- 2 cloves garlic, minced
- 1 teaspoon chopped fresh rosemary
- Salt and pepper to taste
- Chopped fresh parsley for garnish (optional)

Preparation:

1. Steam cauliflower florets until tender, about 10-12 minutes.
2. In a skillet, heat olive oil over medium heat. Add minced garlic and chopped fresh rosemary, and cook until fragrant.
3. Add steamed cauliflower florets and drained chickpeas to the skillet. Cook for 3-4 minutes, stirring occasionally, until heated through.
4. Use a potato masher or fork to mash the cauliflower and chickpeas until desired consistency is reached.
5. Season with salt and pepper to taste.
6. Garnish with chopped fresh parsley before serving if desired.

Nutrition Facts (per serving):

- Calories: 200
- Carbs: 20g
- Protein: 10g
- Fat: 10g

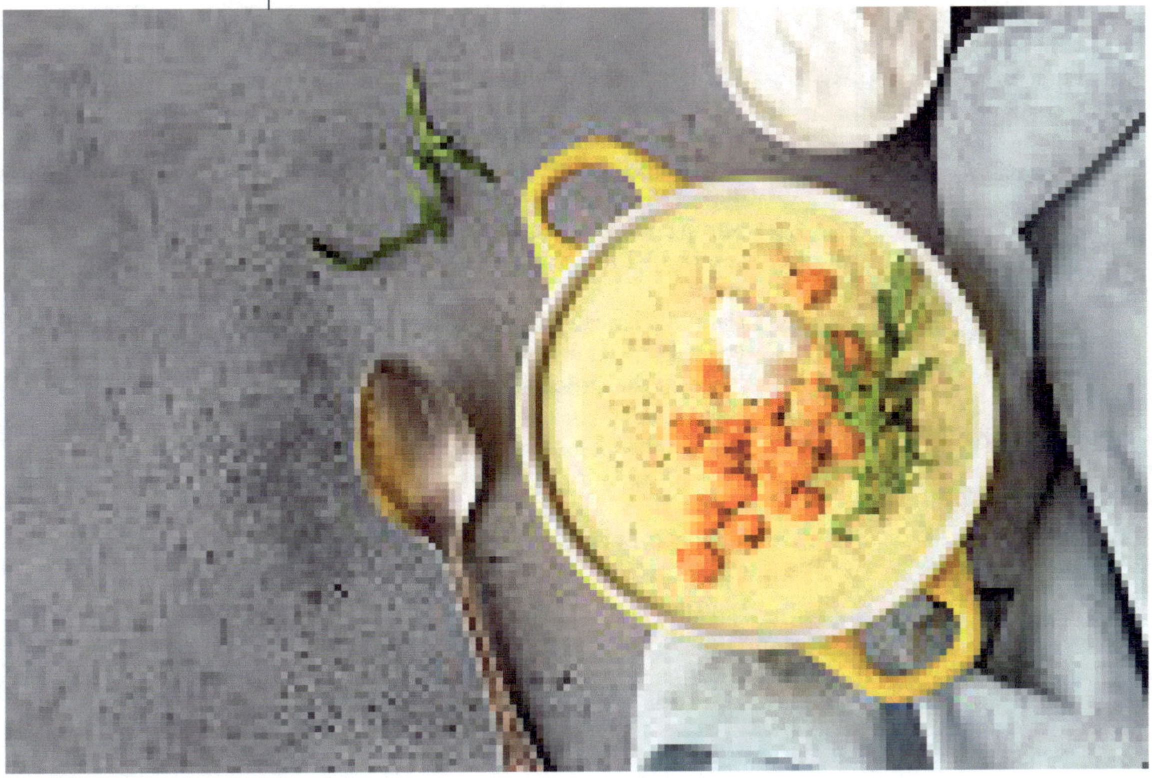

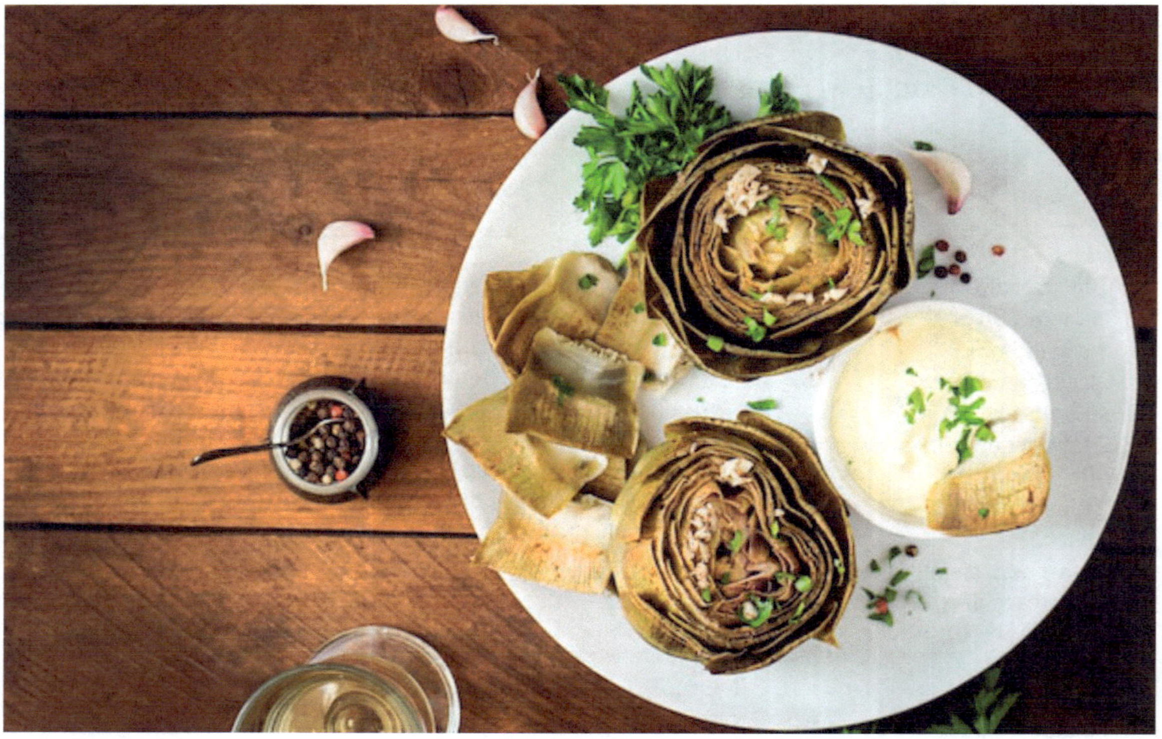

45. Quinoa and Vegetable Stuffed Artichokes

Prep.Time: 20 min

Cook Time: 50 min

Serving: 4

Beverage pairing: Iced Tea

Ingredients:

- 4 large artichokes
- 1 cup cooked quinoa
- 1 small onion, diced
- 1 carrot, diced
- 1 celery stalk, diced
- 1/2 cup diced tomatoes
- 1/4 cup chopped fresh parsley
- 2 tablespoons olive oil
- 2 cloves garlic, minced
- Salt and pepper to taste
- Lemon wedges for serving

Preparation:

1. Trim the stems and top 1/3 of each artichoke. Remove tough outer leaves and trim any sharp tips.
2. In a large pot of boiling water, cook artichokes for 20-30 minutes, or until outer leaves can be easily pulled off. Drain and let cool.
3. Preheat oven to 375°F (190°C).
4. In a skillet, heat olive oil over medium heat. Add diced onion, diced carrot, diced celery, and minced garlic, and sauté until softened.
5. Stir in cooked quinoa, diced tomatoes, and chopped fresh parsley. Cook for another 2-3 minutes until heated through. Season with salt and pepper to taste.
6. Carefully spread apart the leaves of each artichoke and spoon quinoa and vegetable mixture into the center and between the leaves.
7. Place stuffed artichokes in a baking dish and cover with aluminum foil.
8. Bake in the preheated oven for 20-25 minutes, or until heated through.
9. Serve hot with lemon wedges on the side for squeezing.

Nutrition Facts (per serving):

- Calories: 250
- Carbs: 35g
- Protein: 10g
- Fat: 8g

46. Grilled Tofu and Vegetable Wrap with Avocado Cream

Prep.Time: 15 min

Cook Time: 10 min

Serving: 4

Beverage pairing: Herbal Tea

Ingredients:

- 1 block firm tofu, drained and pressed
- 1 tablespoon olive oil
- 1 teaspoon ground cumin
- 1 teaspoon smoked paprika
- Salt and pepper to taste
- 4 large whole wheat or low-carb tortillas
- 1 cup mixed vegetables (bell peppers, onions, zucchini), sliced
- 1 ripe avocado
- Juice of 1 lime
- 2 tablespoons Greek yogurt (unsweetened)

Preparation:

1. Preheat grill to medium-high heat.
2. Slice tofu into thick strips. In a bowl, toss tofu strips with olive oil, ground cumin, smoked paprika, salt, and pepper until well coated.
3. Grill tofu strips for 3-4 minutes per side, or until grill marks appear and tofu is heated through.
4. In the meantime, heat a skillet over medium heat. Add sliced mixed vegetables and sauté until tender.
5. To make the avocado cream, mash the ripe avocado in a bowl. Stir in lime juice, Greek yogurt, salt, and pepper until smooth.
6. Warm tortillas according to package instructions.
7. Spread a generous dollop of avocado cream onto each tortilla.
8. Arrange grilled tofu strips and sautéed mixed vegetables on top of the avocado cream.
9. Roll up the tortillas to form wraps.
10. Serve immediately.

Nutrition Facts (per serving):

- Calories: 300
- Carbs: 25g
- Protein: 12g
- Fat: 18g

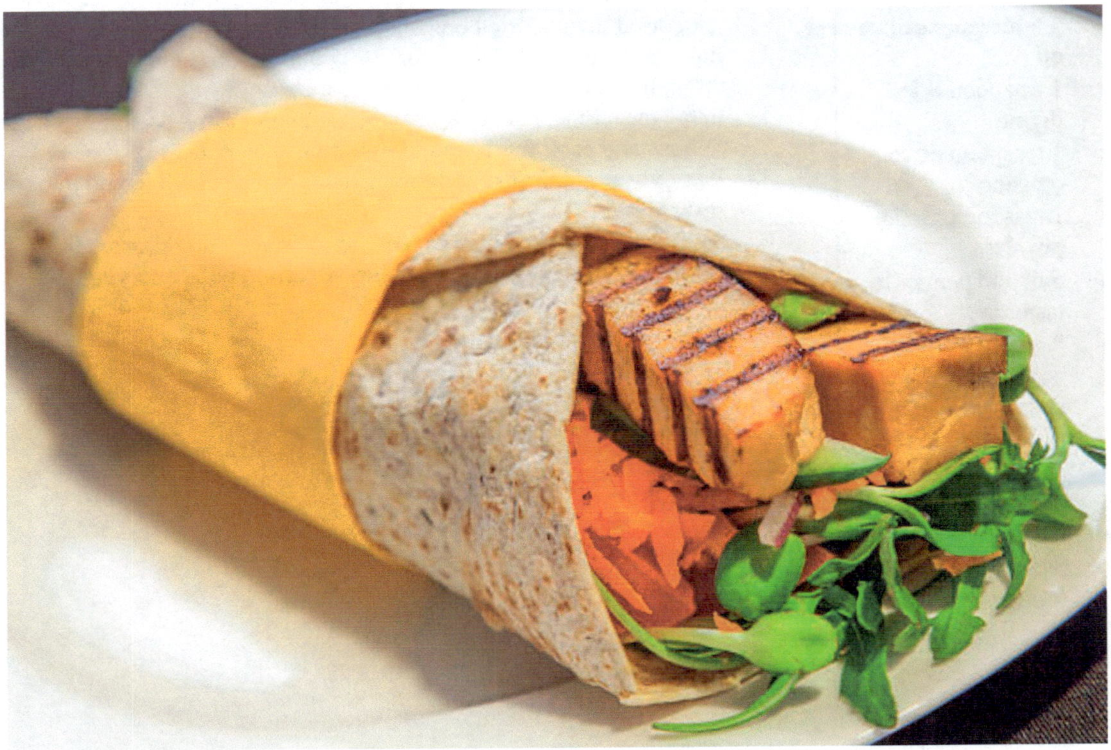

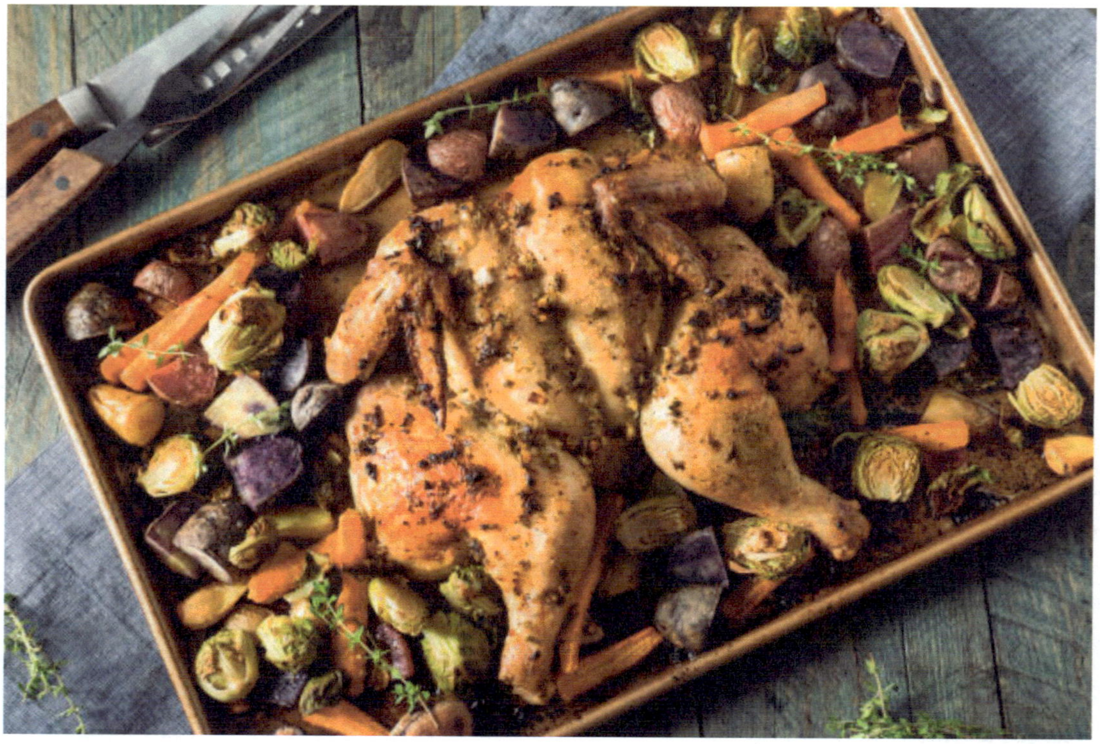

47. Baked Chicken with Herbed Zucchini Ribbons

Prep.Time: 10 min

Cook Time: 25 min

Serving: 4

Beverage pairing: Iced Tea

Ingredients:

- 4 boneless, skinless chicken breasts
- 2 tablespoons olive oil
- 1 teaspoon dried thyme
- 1 teaspoon dried oregano
- 1 teaspoon garlic powder
- Salt and pepper to taste
- 2 medium zucchinis, spiralized into ribbons
- Juice of 1 lemon
- Zest of 1 lemon
- Chopped fresh parsley for garnish (optional)

Preparation:

1. Preheat oven to 375°F (190°C).
2. Place chicken breasts in a baking dish. Drizzle with olive oil and sprinkle with dried thyme, dried oregano, garlic powder, salt, and pepper.
3. Bake in the preheated oven for 20-25 minutes, or until chicken is cooked through and no longer pink in the center.
4. In the meantime, heat a skillet over medium heat. Add spiralized zucchini ribbons and cook for 2-3 minutes until just tender.
5. Remove zucchini ribbons from the heat and toss with lemon juice and lemon zest.
6. Serve baked chicken breasts with herbed zucchini ribbons.
7. Garnish with chopped fresh parsley if desired before serving.

Nutrition Facts (per serving):

- Calories: 250
- Carbs: 6g
- Protein: 30g
- Fat: 12g

48. Spinach and Mushroom Egg Muffins with Feta

Prep.Time: 10 min

Cook Time: 20 min

Serving: 4

Beverage pairing: Black Coffee

Ingredients:

- 8 large eggs
- 1/4 cup milk (unsweetened)
- 1 cup chopped spinach
- 1 cup sliced mushrooms
- 1/4 cup crumbled feta cheese
- Salt and pepper to taste
- Cooking spray

Preparation:

1. Preheat oven to 350°F (175°C). Grease a muffin tin with cooking spray.
2. In a bowl, whisk together eggs and milk until well combined.
3. Stir in chopped spinach, sliced mushrooms, crumbled feta cheese, salt, and pepper.
4. Divide the egg mixture evenly among the muffin cups.
5. Bake in the preheated oven for 20-25 minutes, or until egg muffins are set and lightly golden on top.
6. Remove from oven and let cool slightly before serving.
7. Store leftovers in an airtight container in the refrigerator for up to 3 days.

Nutrition Facts (per serving, serving size: 2 egg muffins):

- Calories: 200
- Carbs: 3g
- Protein: 15g
- Fat: 14g

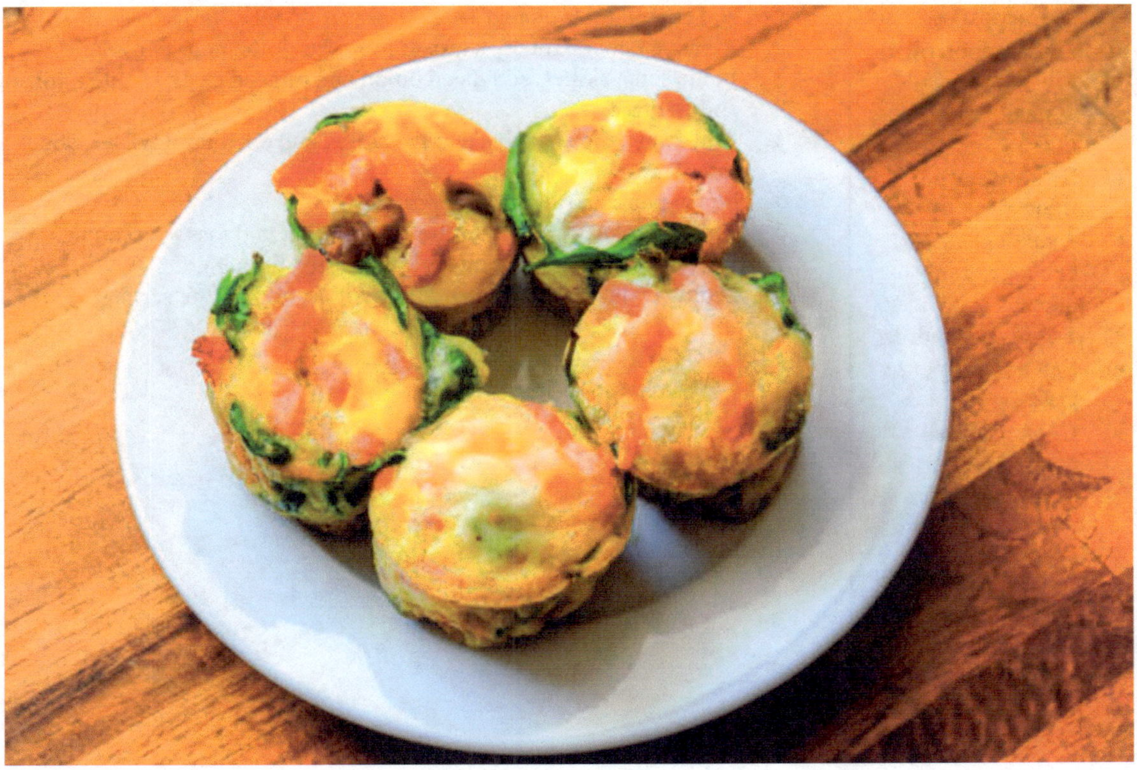

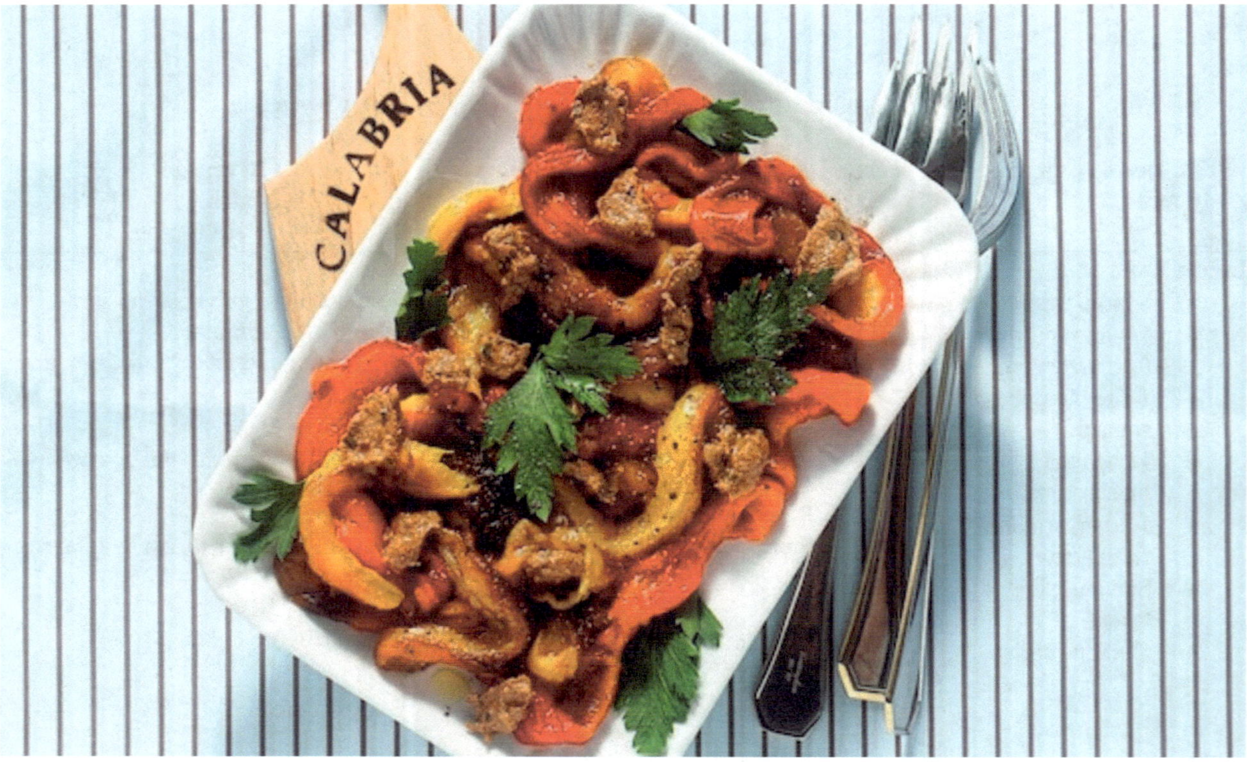

49. Cabbage and Turkey Sausage Skillet with Paprika

Prep.Time: 10 min

Cook Time: 15 min

Serving: 4

Beverage pairing: Iced Tea

Ingredients:

- 1 pound turkey sausage, sliced
- 1 tablespoon olive oil
- 1 small onion, diced
- 2 cloves garlic, minced
- 1 small head cabbage, thinly sliced
- 1 teaspoon paprika
- Salt and pepper to taste
- Chopped fresh parsley for garnish (optional)

Preparation:

1. In a large skillet, heat olive oil over medium heat. Add sliced turkey sausage and cook until browned.
2. Remove cooked turkey sausage from the skillet and set aside.
3. In the same skillet, add diced onion and minced garlic. Sauté until softened and fragrant.
4. Add thinly sliced cabbage to the skillet and cook until wilted, about 5-7 minutes.
5. Stir in paprika, salt, and pepper.
6. Return cooked turkey sausage to the skillet and toss to combine.
7. Cook for another 2-3 minutes until heated through.
8. Garnish with chopped fresh parsley if desired before serving.

Nutrition Facts (per serving):

- Calories: 300
- Carbs: 10g
- Protein: 20g
- Fat: 20g

50. Zoodle (Zucchini Noodle) Primavera with Grilled Chicken

Prep.Time: 15 min

Cook Time: 15 min

Serving: 4

Beverage pairing: Herbal Tea

Ingredients:

- 4 boneless, skinless chicken breasts
- 2 tablespoons olive oil
- Salt and pepper to taste
- 4 medium zucchinis, spiralized into noodles
- 1 cup cherry tomatoes, halved
- 1 cup sliced bell peppers
- 1/2 cup sliced mushrooms
- 2 cloves garlic, minced
- 1/4 cup chopped fresh basil
- Juice of 1 lemon

Preparation:

1. Preheat grill to medium-high heat.
2. Brush chicken breasts with olive oil and season with salt and pepper.
3. Grill chicken for 6-8 minutes per side, or until cooked through. Let rest for a few minutes before slicing.
4. In the meantime, heat olive oil in a large skillet over medium heat. Add minced garlic and cook until fragrant.
5. Add spiralized zucchini noodles, halved cherry tomatoes, sliced bell peppers, and sliced mushrooms to the skillet. Cook for 3-4 minutes until vegetables are tender-crisp.
6. Stir in chopped fresh basil and lemon juice. Cook for another minute.
7. Divide zoodle primavera among serving plates and top with sliced grilled chicken.
8. Serve hot, optionally sprinkled with grated Parmesan cheese.

Nutrition Facts (per serving):

- Calories: 250
- Carbs: 10g
- Protein: 30g
- Fat: 10g

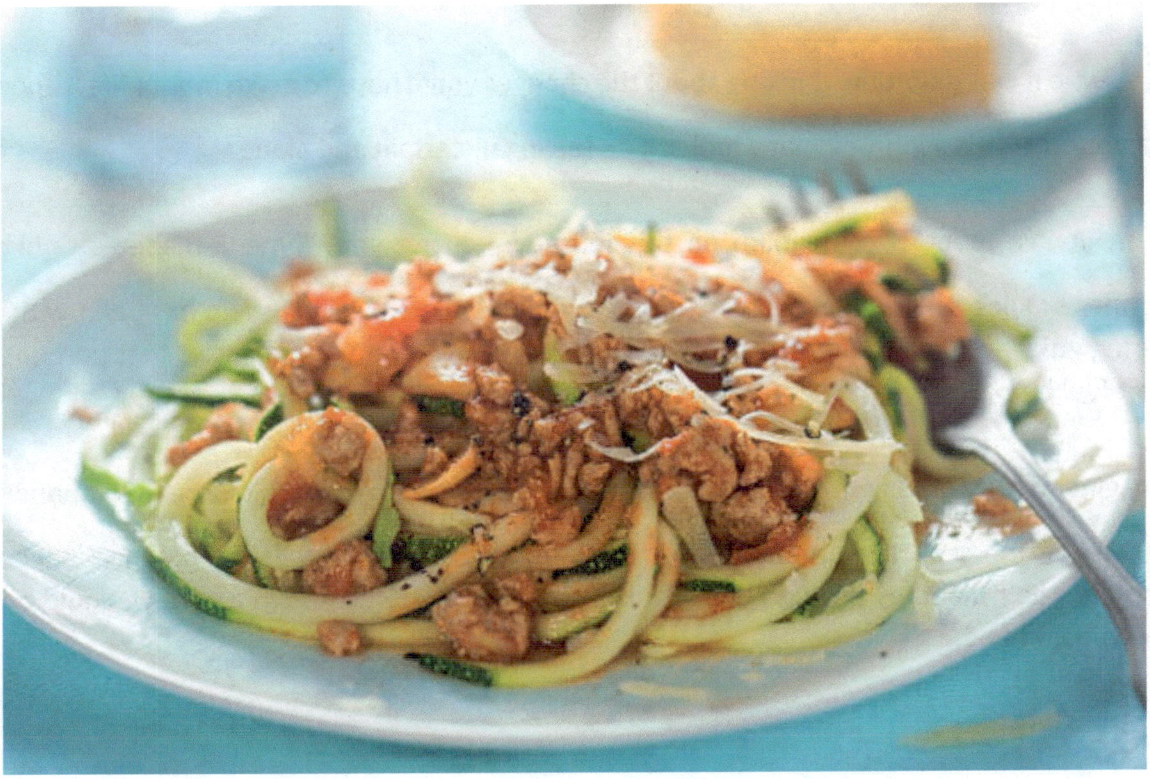

Your Kindness is Key

Share Your Experience, Share Your Strength

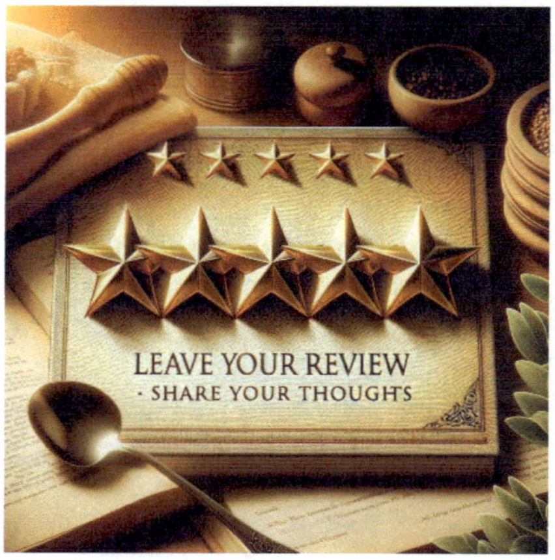

"Helping one person might not change the whole world, but it could change the world for one person." - Anonymous

Do you remember what it was like when you first heard the words "Type 2 Diabetes?" Perhaps it felt like a mountain you weren't sure you could climb.

Maybe it was daunting, thinking about the changes you'd have to make in your life, especially with your diet. It's a journey many embark on feeling uncertain and alone.

But you've found a companion on this journey, haven't you? Type 2 Diabetes Cookbook Beginner's Quick & Easy Recipes for Delicious Diabetes Diets by Lily Anders has been with you, offering guidance, delicious recipes, and a sense of control over your diabetes that perhaps you didn't feel before.

Imagine if you could light the path for someone just starting on this journey. Someone who feels lost in the sea of information, unsure of where to turn for reliable, practical advice on managing their diabetes through diet. Your experience, shared through a review, could be the beacon they need.

This isn't just about leaving a review; it's about extending a hand, offering support, and sharing the strength that comes from knowledge and community. Your words could help another person find their footing, making their journey a bit easier and less lonely.

So, here's my humble request on behalf of a fellow journeyer you've yet to meet:

Please take a moment to share your experience with the book. Your insights could be the very thing another person needs to hear to take that first, brave step toward a healthier, happier life with diabetes. Your review, a simple act of kindness, asks for nothing in return yet offers immeasurable value.

To leave your review, just follow this link:

https://www.amazon.com/review/create-review/?ie=UTF8&channel=glance-detail&asin=1963939336

If the thought of helping another soul on their diabetes journey warms your heart, then you're exactly who I hoped to reach with this book. Welcome to a community where kindness, support, and shared victories pave the way to a better life.

I'm beyond grateful for your help in spreading the word and even more excited to continue providing you with the knowledge and recipes to make managing diabetes not just manageable, but enjoyable.

Click the QR Code Here!

Thank you from the deepest places in my heart. Your generosity makes all the difference.

Lily Anders

P.S. - Sharing is caring, they say. If you believe this book has brought value to your life and could do the same for someone else, consider sharing it with them. It's another beautiful way to change a life, one meal at a time.

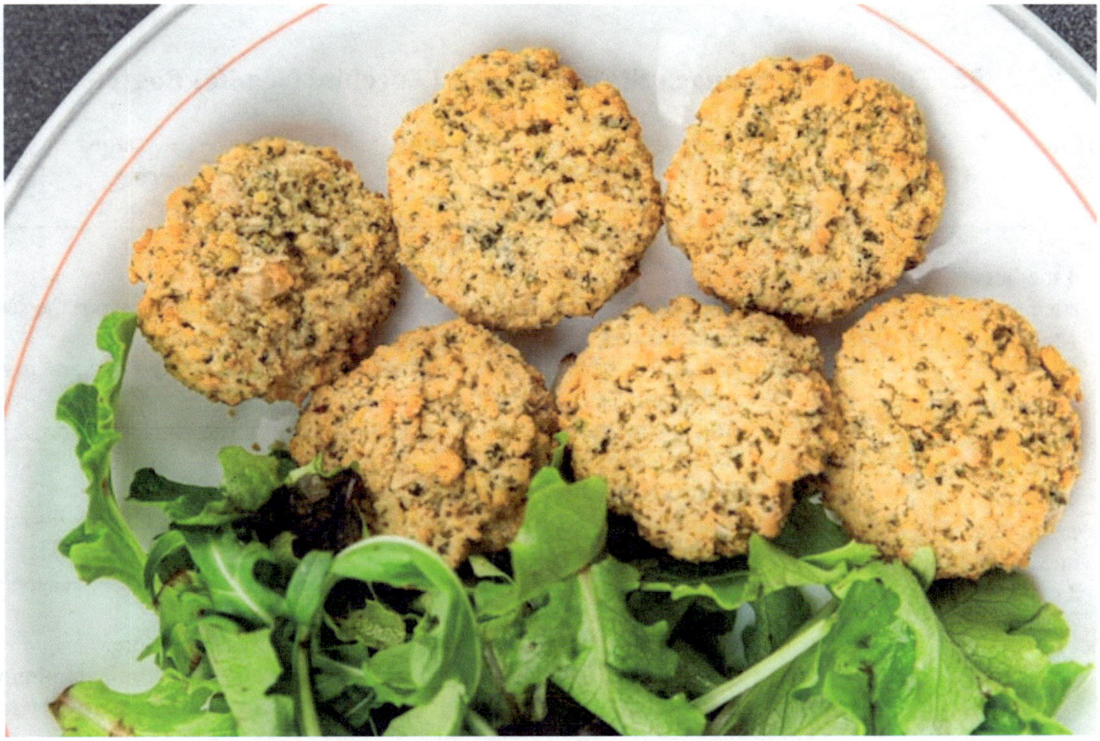

51. Cauliflower and Chickpea Patties with Avocado Mayo

Prep.Time: 15 min

Cook Time: 10 min

Serving: 4

Beverage pairing: Iced Tea

Ingredients:

- 1 cup cooked cauliflower florets
- 1 can (15 oz) chickpeas, drained and rinsed
- 1/4 cup almond flour
- 1/4 cup chopped fresh cilantro
- 2 cloves garlic, minced
- 1 teaspoon ground cumin
- 1/2 teaspoon paprika
- Salt and pepper to taste
- 2 tablespoons olive oil
- 1 ripe avocado
- 2 tablespoons Greek yogurt (unsweetened)

Preparation:

1. In a food processor, pulse together cooked cauliflower florets and chickpeas until coarsely mashed.
2. Transfer the mixture to a bowl. Add almond flour, chopped fresh cilantro, minced garlic, ground cumin, paprika, salt, and pepper. Mix until well combined.
3. Form the mixture into patties.
4. In a skillet, heat olive oil over medium heat. Cook the patties for 3-4 minutes per side, or until golden brown and heated through.
5. Meanwhile, prepare the avocado mayo by mashing the ripe avocado in a bowl. Stir in Greek yogurt and lemon juice until smooth. Season with salt and pepper to taste.
6. Serve the cauliflower and chickpea patties with avocado mayo on the side.

Nutrition Facts (per serving, serving size: 2 patties with avocado mayo):

- Calories: 300
- Carbs: 20g
- Protein: 10g
- Fat: 20g

52. Turkey and Spinach Stuffed Zoodle (Zucchini Noodle) Boats

Prep.Time: 20 min

Cook Time: 25 min

Serving: 4

Beverage pairing: Herbal Tea

Ingredients:

- 4 medium zucchinis
- 1 tablespoon olive oil
- 1 small onion, diced
- 1 clove garlic, minced
- 1 pound ground turkey
- 2 cups chopped fresh spinach
- 1/4 cup grated Parmesan cheese
- Salt and pepper to taste

Preparation:

1. Preheat oven to 375°F (190°C).
2. Cut each zucchini in half lengthwise. Use a spoon to scoop out the seeds and flesh, leaving a boat-shaped shell. Reserve the flesh for later use.
3. In a skillet, heat olive oil over medium heat. Add diced onion and minced garlic, and sauté until softened.
4. Add ground turkey to the skillet and cook until browned, breaking it into small pieces as it cooks.
5. Stir in chopped fresh spinach and cook until wilted.
6. Chop the reserved zucchini flesh and add it to the skillet. Cook for another 2-3 minutes.
7. Remove skillet from heat and stir in grated Parmesan cheese. Season with salt and pepper to taste.
8. Fill each zucchini boat with the turkey and spinach mixture.
9. Place stuffed zucchini boats in a baking dish and cover with aluminum foil.
10. Bake in the preheated oven for 20-25 minutes, or until zucchini is tender.
11. Serve hot.

Nutrition Facts (per serving):

- Calories: 250
- Carbs: 10g
- Protein: 30g
- Fat: 10g

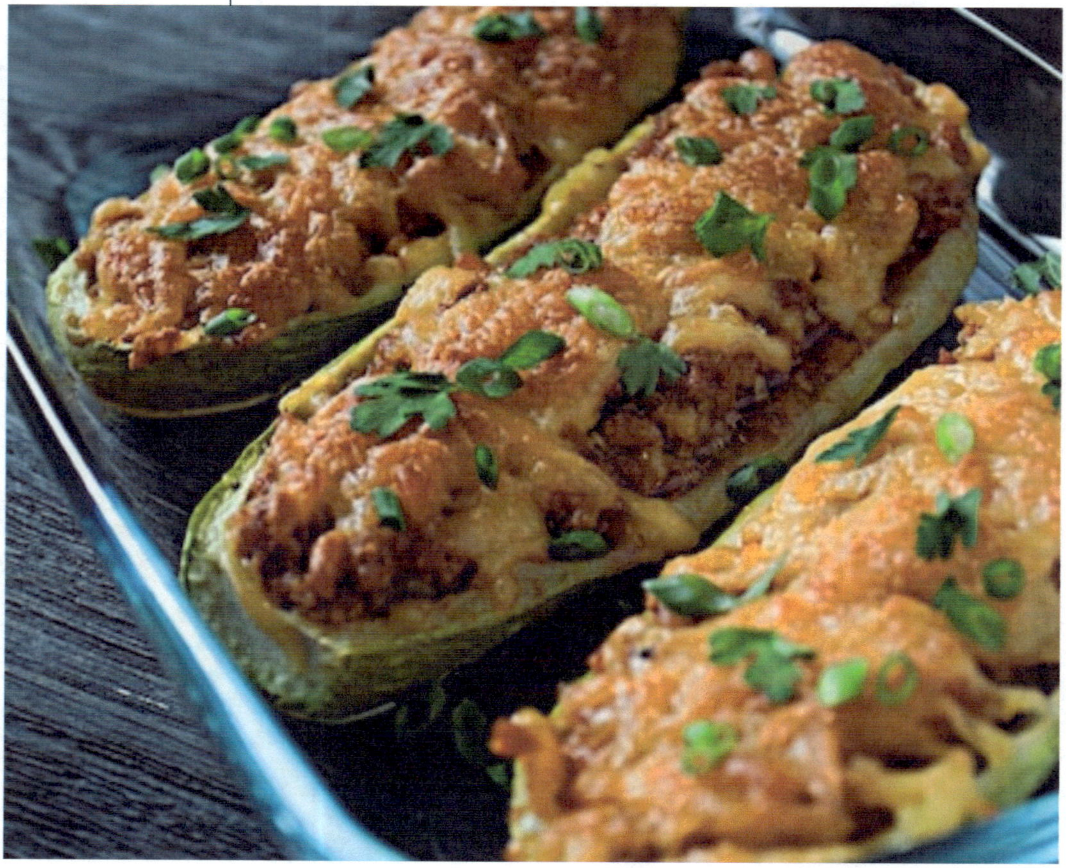

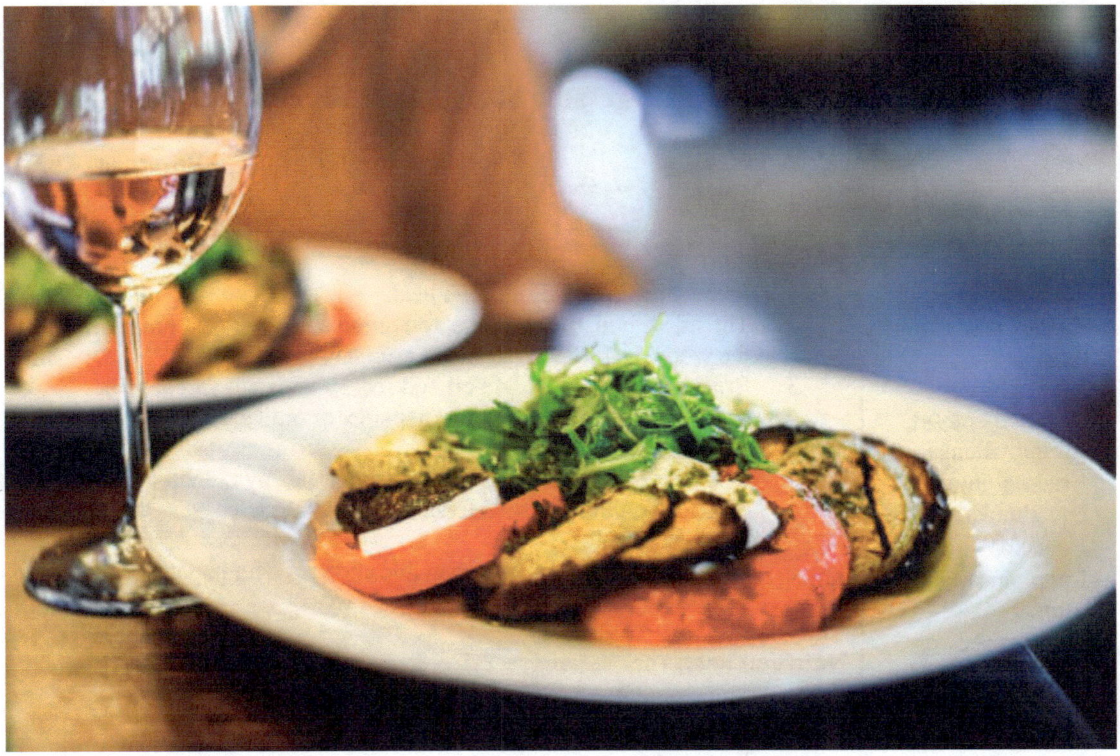

53. Eggplant and Tomato Caprese with Balsamic Glaze

Prep.Time: 15 min

Cook Time: 6 min

Serving: 4

Beverage pairing: Iced Tea

Ingredients:

- 1 large eggplant
- 2 large tomatoes
- 8 ounces fresh mozzarella cheese, cut into cubes
- Fresh basil leaves
- Balsamic glaze (store-bought or homemade)
- Wooden skewers, soaked in water for 30 minutes

Preparation:

1. Preheat grill or grill pan over medium-high heat.
2. Cut eggplant and tomatoes into slices.
3. Thread eggplant slices, tomato slices, fresh mozzarella cubes, and basil leaves onto the wooden skewers, alternating the ingredients.
4. Grill skewers for 2-3 minutes per side, or until grill marks appear and vegetables are tender.
5. Arrange grilled skewers on a serving platter.
6. Drizzle with balsamic glaze before serving.

Nutrition Facts (per serving, serving size: 2 skewers):

- Calories: 200
- Carbs: 10g
- Protein: 12g
- Fat: 14g

54. Grilled Shrimp and Vegetable Skewers with Pineapple Salsa

Prep.Time: 20 min

Cook Time: 6 min

Serving: 4

Beverage pairing: Herbal Tea

Ingredients:

- 1 pound large shrimp, peeled and deveined
- 2 bell peppers (assorted colors), cut into chunks
- 1 red onion, cut into chunks
- 1 zucchini, sliced
- 1 cup pineapple chunks
- Wooden skewers, soaked in water for 30 minutes
- Olive oil for brushing
- Salt and pepper to taste

Preparation:

1. Preheat grill to medium-high heat.
2. Thread shrimp, bell peppers, red onion, zucchini, and pineapple chunks onto the wooden skewers, alternating the ingredients.
3. Brush skewers with olive oil and season with salt and pepper.
4. Grill skewers for 2-3 minutes per side, or until shrimp are pink and vegetables are tender.
5. In the meantime, prepare the pineapple salsa by combining diced pineapple, diced red onion, chopped fresh cilantro, lime juice, salt, and pepper in a bowl. Mix well.
6. Serve grilled shrimp and vegetable skewers with pineapple salsa on the side.

Nutrition Facts (per serving, serving size: 2 skewers with salsa):

- Calories: 250
- Carbs: 15g
- Protein: 25g
- Fat: 10g

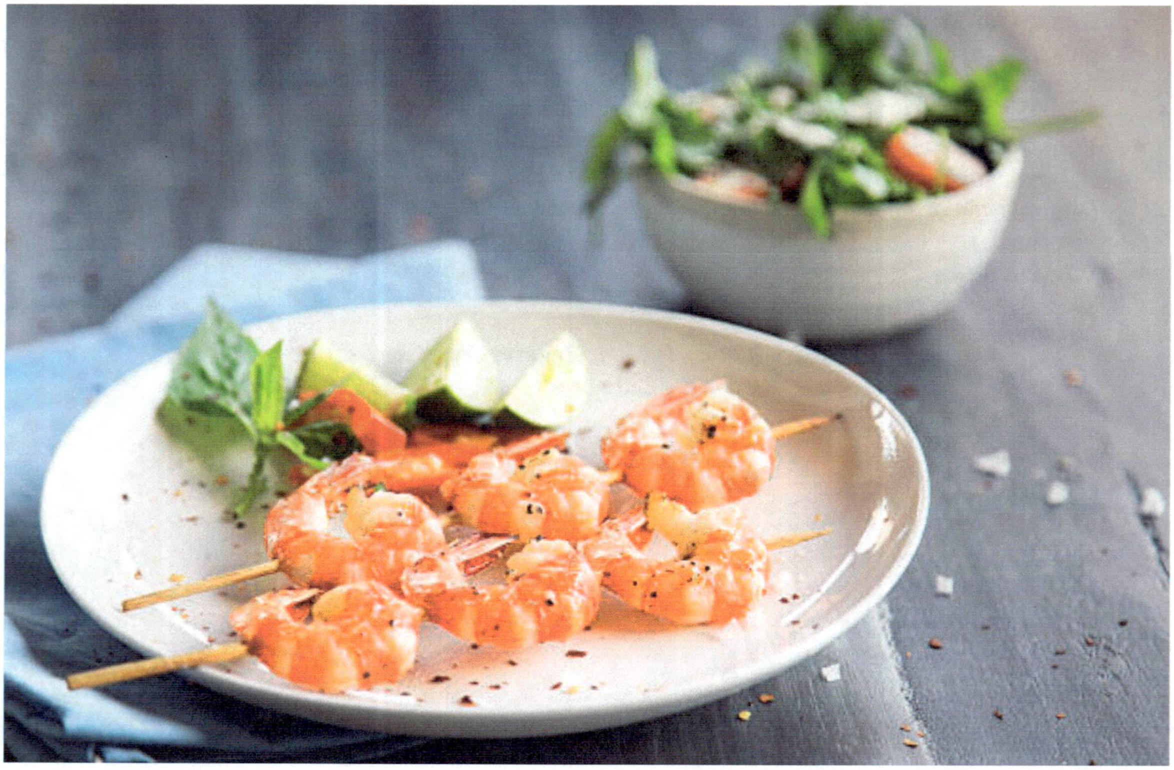

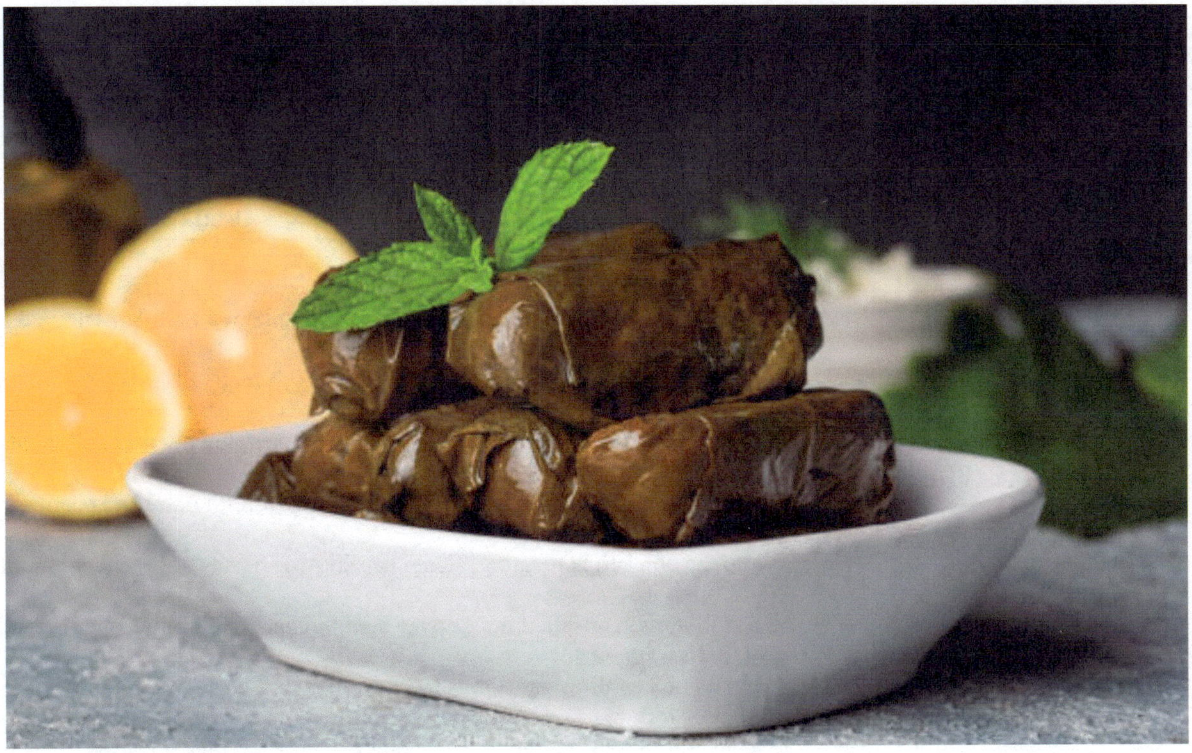

55. Mediterranean Turkey and Quinoa Stuffed Grape Leaves

Prep.Time: 30 min

Cook Time: 25 min

Serving: 4

Beverage pairing: Iced Tea

Ingredients:

- 1 jar grape leaves in brine, drained and rinsed
- 1 cup cooked quinoa
- 1 pound ground turkey
- 1 small onion, finely chopped
- 2 cloves garlic, minced
- 1/4 cup chopped fresh parsley
- 1 teaspoon dried oregano
- Juice of 1 lemon
- Salt and pepper to taste
- Olive oil for brushing

Preparation:

1. Preheat oven to 350°F (175°C).
2. In a skillet, heat olive oil over medium heat. Add chopped onion and minced garlic, and sauté until softened.
3. Add ground turkey to the skillet and cook until browned, breaking it into small pieces as it cooks.
4. Stir in cooked quinoa, chopped fresh parsley, dried oregano, lemon juice, salt, and pepper. Cook for another 2-3 minutes until heated through.
5. Remove skillet from heat and let the mixture cool slightly.
6. Place a grape leaf on a flat surface, shiny side down. Spoon a small amount of the turkey and quinoa mixture onto the center of the grape leaf.
7. Fold the sides of the grape leaf over the filling, then roll up tightly.
8. Repeat with the remaining grape leaves and filling.
9. Place stuffed grape leaves in a baking dish, seam side down.
10. Brush the tops of the stuffed grape leaves with olive oil.
11. Bake in the preheated oven for 20-25 minutes, or until heated through.
12. Serve warm.

Nutrition Facts (per serving, serving size: 4 stuffed grape leaves):

- Calories: 300
- Carbs: 20g
- Protein: 25g
- Fat: 12g

56. Lemon Garlic Chicken Thighs with Cauliflower Mash

Prep.Time: 15 min

Cook Time: 30 min

Serving: 4

Beverage pairing: Iced Tea

Ingredients:

- 4 bone-in, skin-on chicken thighs
- 2 tablespoons olive oil
- 2 cloves garlic, minced
- Zest and juice of 1 lemon
- 1 teaspoon dried thyme
- Salt and pepper to taste
- 1 head cauliflower, cut into florets
- 2 cloves garlic, minced
- 2 tablespoons unsalted butter

Preparation:

1. Preheat oven to 400°F (200°C).
2. In a bowl, mix together olive oil, minced garlic, lemon zest, lemon juice, dried thyme, salt, and pepper.
3. Pat chicken thighs dry with paper towels and rub them with the lemon garlic mixture.
4. Place chicken thighs skin-side up on a baking sheet lined with parchment paper.
5. Roast in the preheated oven for 25-30 minutes, or until chicken is cooked through and skin is crispy.
6. While the chicken is roasting, steam cauliflower florets until tender, about 10-12 minutes.
7. In a skillet, melt unsalted butter over medium heat. Add minced garlic and cook until fragrant.
8. Add steamed cauliflower florets to the skillet and mash them with a potato masher or fork until smooth. Season cauliflower mash with salt and pepper to taste. Serve roasted lemon garlic chicken thighs with cauliflower mash.
9. Garnish with chopped fresh parsley if desired before serving.

Nutrition Facts (per serving):

- Calories: 350
- Carbs: 10g
- Protein: 25g
- Fat: 25g

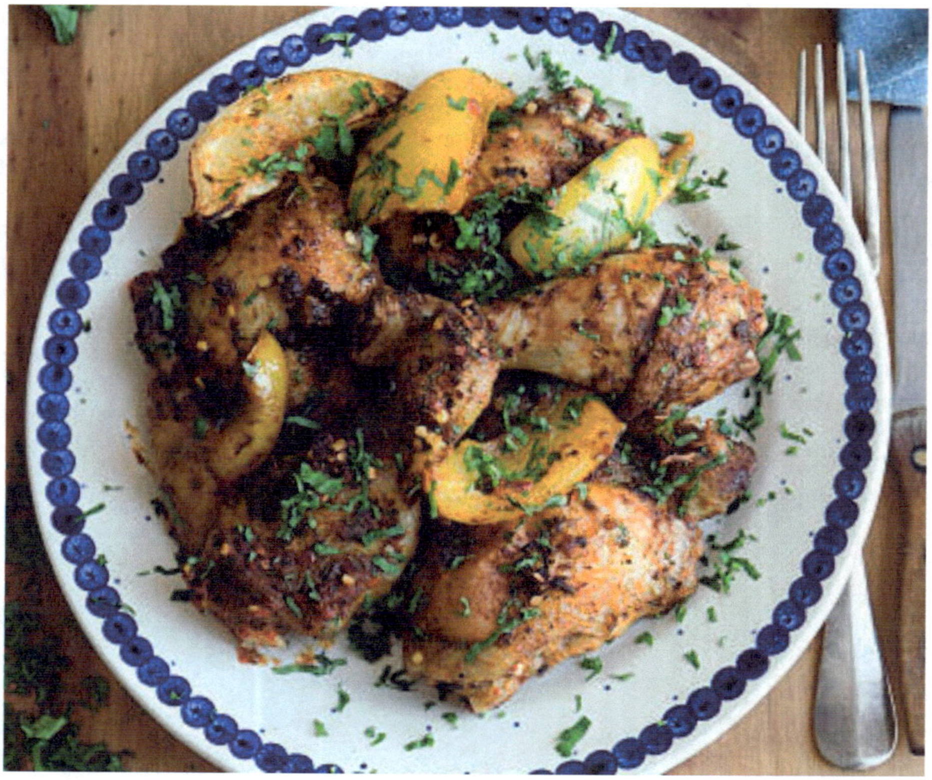

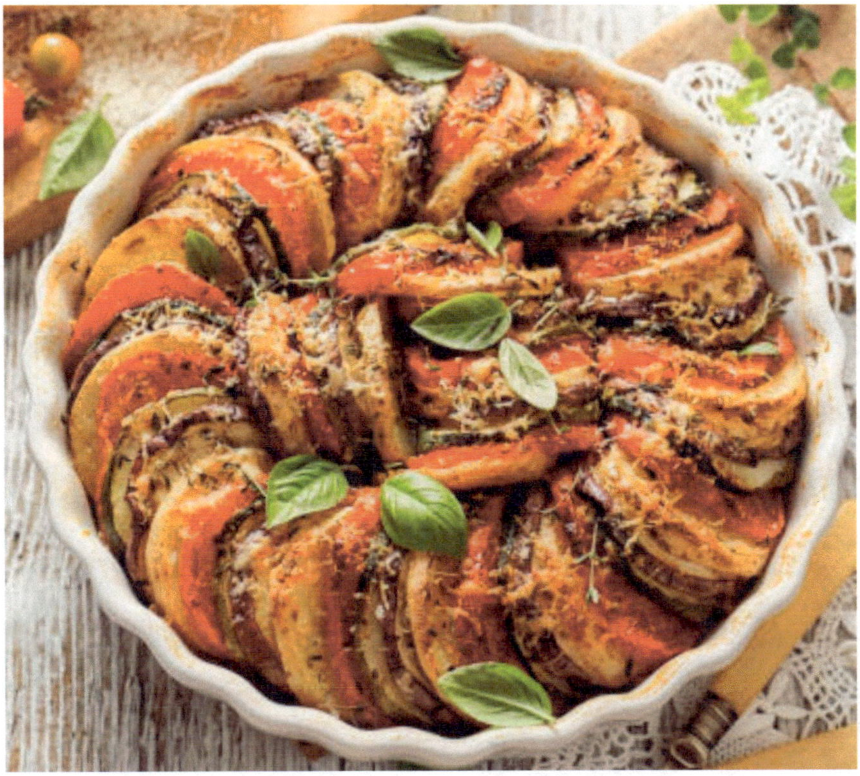

57. Zucchini and Tomato Tian with Herbed Breadcrumbs

Prep.Time: 15 min

Cook Time: 35 min

Serving: 4

Beverage pairing: Herbal Tea

Ingredients:

- 2 large zucchinis, sliced into rounds
- 2 large tomatoes, sliced into rounds
- 2 cloves garlic, minced
- 2 tablespoons olive oil
- Salt and pepper to taste
- 1 cup breadcrumbs (whole wheat or low-carb)
- 2 tablespoons chopped fresh parsley
- 1 tablespoon chopped fresh thyme
- 1 tablespoon olive oil

Preparation:

1. Preheat oven to 375°F (190°C).
2. In a bowl, toss zucchini rounds and tomato rounds with minced garlic, olive oil, salt, and pepper until well coated.
3. Arrange zucchini and tomato rounds in overlapping layers in a baking dish.
4. In a separate bowl, mix together breadcrumbs, chopped fresh parsley, chopped fresh thyme, olive oil, salt, and pepper.
5. Sprinkle the herbed breadcrumbs mixture evenly over the zucchini and tomato layers.
6. Cover the baking dish with aluminum foil and bake in the preheated oven for 20 minutes.
7. Remove foil and bake for an additional 10-15 minutes, or until breadcrumbs are golden brown and vegetables are tender.
8. Serve hot.

Nutrition Facts (per serving):

- Calories: 200
- Carbs: 20g
- Protein: 5g
- Fat: 10g

58. Cauliflower and Chickpea Tandoori with Raita

Prep.Time: 10 min

Cook Time: 30 min

Serving: 4

Beverage pairing: Iced Tea

Ingredients:

- 1 head cauliflower, cut into florets
- 1 can (15 oz) chickpeas, drained and rinsed
- 2 tablespoons olive oil
- 2 tablespoons Tandoori seasoning
- Salt to taste
- 1 cup plain Greek yogurt (unsweetened)
- 1/2 cucumber, grated and squeezed to remove excess moisture
- 1/4 cup chopped fresh mint
- 1/4 teaspoon ground cumin

Preparation:

1. Preheat oven to 400°F (200°C).
2. In a large bowl, toss cauliflower florets and chickpeas with olive oil, Tandoori seasoning, and salt until well coated.
3. Spread cauliflower and chickpea mixture in a single layer on a baking sheet lined with parchment paper.
4. Roast in the preheated oven for 25-30 minutes, or until cauliflower is tender and chickpeas are crispy.
5. In the meantime, prepare the raita by mixing together plain Greek yogurt, grated cucumber, chopped fresh mint, ground cumin, and salt in a bowl. Stir well to combine.
6. Serve roasted cauliflower and chickpeas with raita on the side.

Nutrition Facts (per serving):

- Calories: 250
- Carbs: 20g
- Protein: 10g
- Fat: 15g

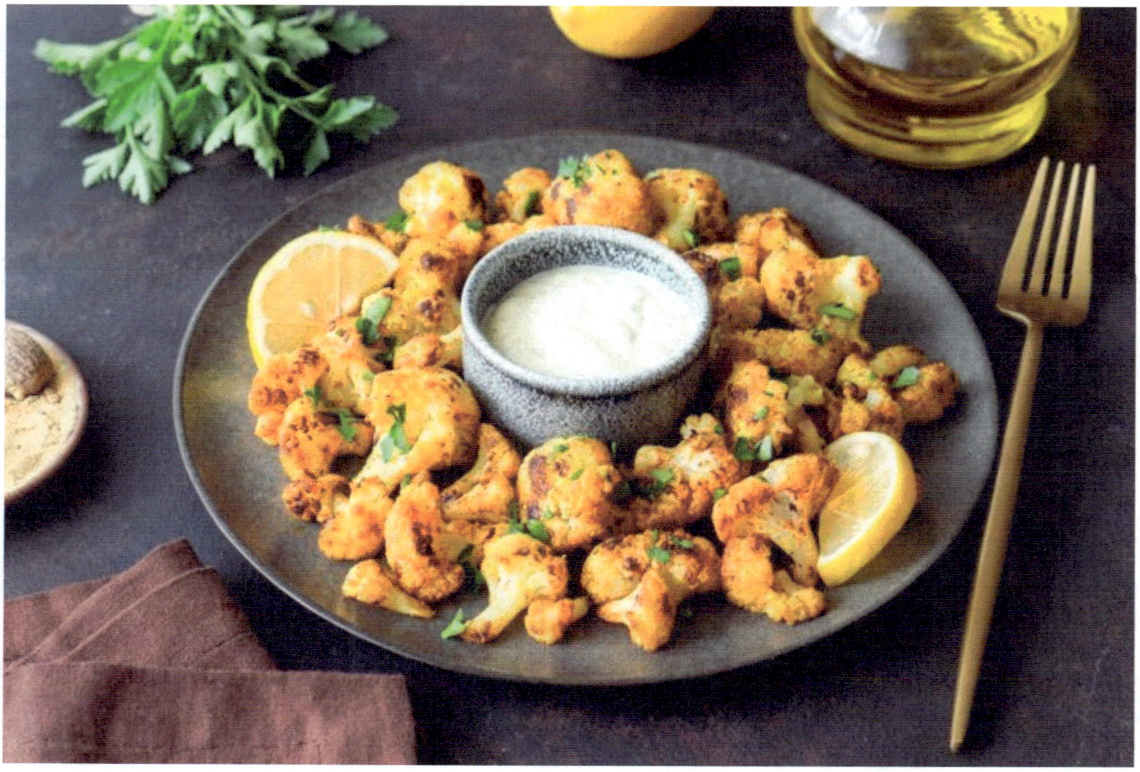

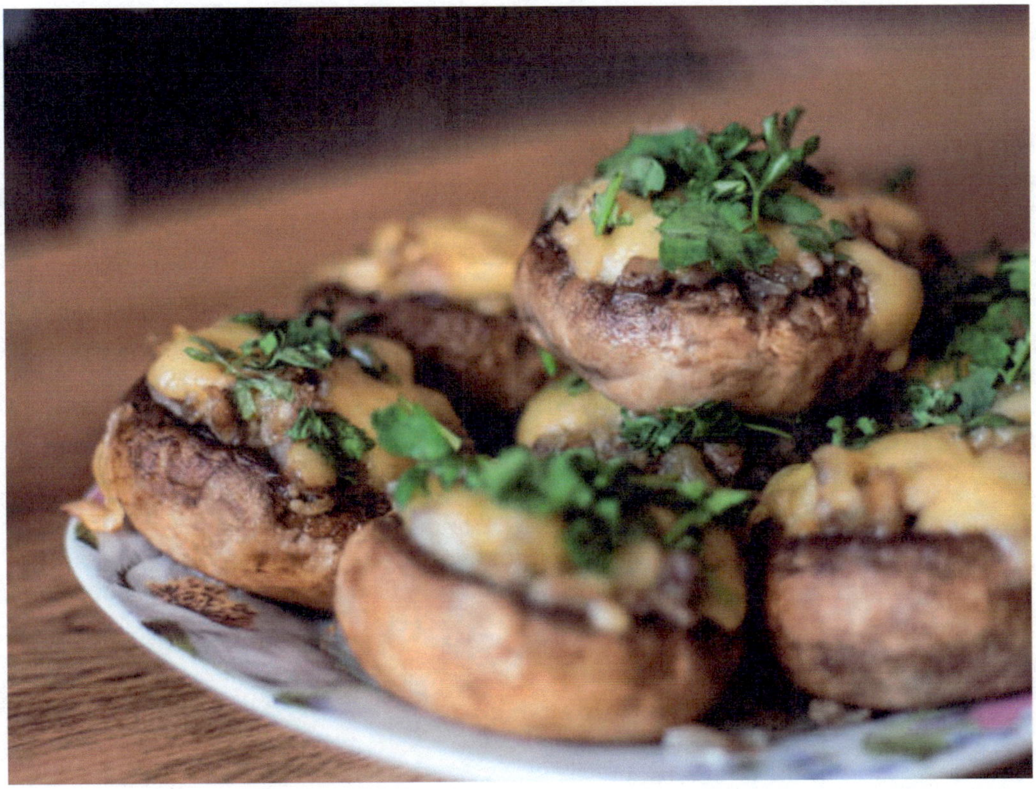

59. Turkey and Spinach Stuffed Portobello Mushroom Caps

Prep.Time: 15 min

Cook Time: 25 min

Serving: 4

Beverage pairing: Herbal Tea

Ingredients:

- 4 large Portobello mushroom caps
- 1 pound ground turkey
- 2 cups chopped fresh spinach
- 1 small onion, diced
- 2 cloves garlic, minced
- 1/4 cup grated Parmesan cheese
- Salt and pepper to taste
- Olive oil for brushing

Preparation:

1. Preheat oven to 375°F (190°C).
2. Remove stems from Portobello mushroom caps and gently scrape out the gills with a spoon.
3. In a skillet, heat olive oil over medium heat. Add diced onion and minced garlic, and sauté until softened.
4. Add ground turkey to the skillet and cook until browned, breaking it into small pieces as it cooks.
5. Stir in chopped fresh spinach and cook until wilted.
6. Remove skillet from heat and stir in grated Parmesan cheese. Season with salt and pepper to taste.
7. Spoon the turkey and spinach mixture into the Portobello mushroom caps.
8. Place stuffed mushroom caps on a baking sheet lined with parchment paper.
9. Brush the tops of the stuffed mushroom caps with olive oil.
10. Bake in the preheated oven for 20-25 minutes, or until mushrooms are tender and filling is heated through.
11. Serve hot.

Nutrition Facts (per serving):

- Calories: 200
- Carbs: 5g
- Protein: 25g
- Fat: 10g

60. Shrimp and Avocado Spring Roll with Peanut Sauce

Prep.Time: 20 min

Cook Time: 5 min

Serving: 4

Beverage pairing: Iced Tea

Ingredients:

- 1 pound large shrimp, peeled and deveined
- 2 tablespoons olive oil
- 4 cups mixed salad greens
- 2 cucumbers, julienned
- 2 carrots, julienned
- 1 avocado, sliced
- 1/4 cup chopped fresh cilantro
- 1/4 cup chopped peanuts
- 1/4 cup natural peanut butter (unsweetened)
- 2 tablespoons soy sauce (reduced-sodium)
- 1 tablespoon rice vinegar
- a sugar-free sweetener
- 1 clove garlic, minced

Preparation:

1. In a skillet, heat olive oil over medium heat. Add shrimp and cook for 2-3 minutes per side, or until pink and cooked through. Remove from heat and set aside.
2. In a small bowl, whisk together natural peanut butter, soy sauce, rice vinegar, honey, minced garlic, and water (as needed to thin out the sauce) until smooth.
3. Arrange mixed salad greens, julienned cucumbers, julienned carrots, sliced avocado, and cooked shrimp in serving bowls.
4. Drizzle peanut sauce over the top of each bowl.
5. Garnish with chopped fresh cilantro and chopped peanuts before serving.

Nutrition Facts (per serving):

- Calories: 350
- Carbs: 15g
- Protein: 25g
- Fat: 25g

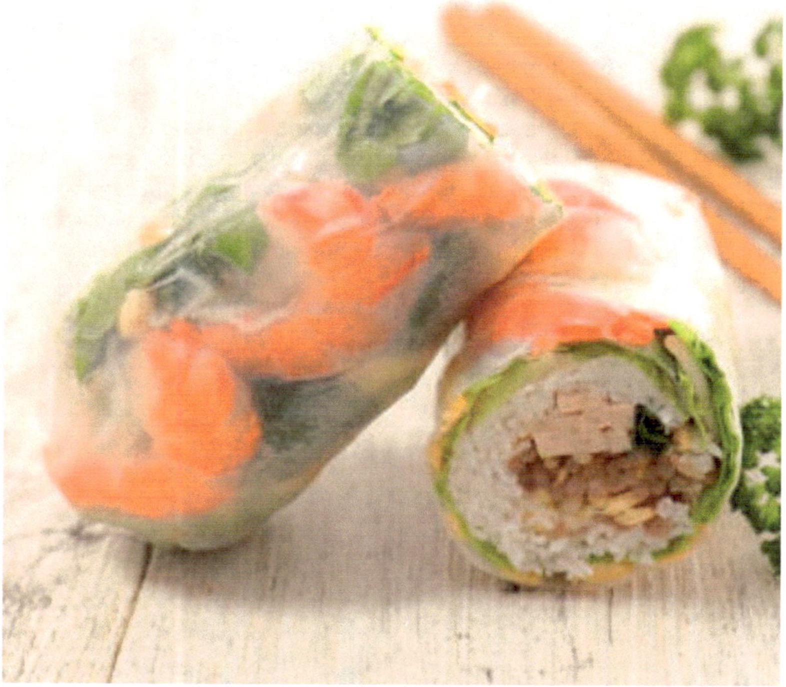

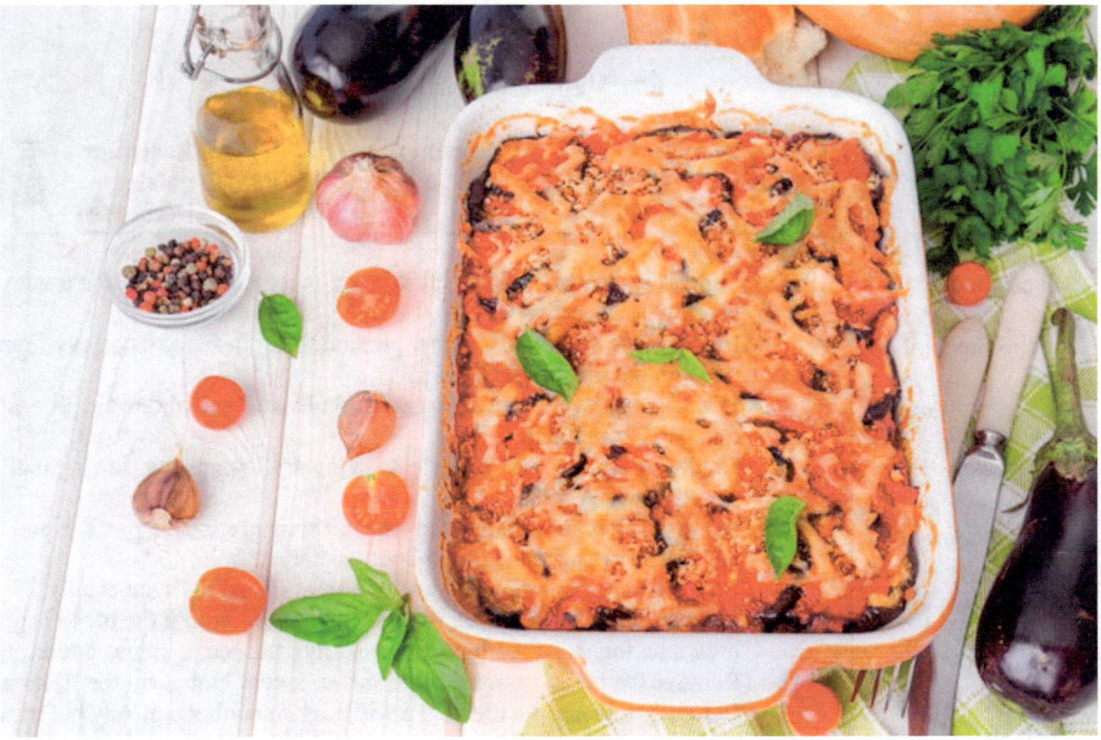

61. Eggplant and Zucchini Lasagna with Turkey and Ricotta

Prep.Time: 30 min | **Cook Time:** 45 min | **Serving:** 6 | **Beverage pairing:** Herbal Tea

Ingredients:

- 1 large eggplant, sliced lengthwise
- 2 medium zucchinis, sliced lengthwise
- 1 pound ground turkey
- 1 small onion, diced
- 2 cloves garlic, minced
- 1 can (15 oz) crushed tomatoes
- 1 teaspoon dried basil
- 1 teaspoon dried oregano
- Salt and pepper to taste
- 1 cup part-skim ricotta cheese
- 1/4 cup grated Parmesan cheese

Preparation:

1. Preheat oven to 375°F (190°C).
2. In a skillet, cook ground turkey over medium heat until browned. Add diced onion and minced garlic, and cook until softened.
3. Stir in crushed tomatoes, dried basil, dried oregano, salt, and pepper. Simmer for 10-15 minutes.
4. In the meantime, lightly grill or roast eggplant and zucchini slices until tender.
5. In a baking dish, layer grilled eggplant and zucchini slices with turkey tomato sauce and dollops of ricotta cheese.
6. Repeat the layers until all ingredients are used, ending with a layer of sauce and a sprinkle of grated Parmesan cheese on top.
7. Cover the baking dish with aluminum foil and bake in the preheated oven for 25-30 minutes.
8. Remove foil and bake for an additional 10 minutes, or until lasagna is bubbly and golden on top.
9. Let the lasagna rest for a few minutes before slicing.
10. Garnish with fresh basil leaves if desired before serving.

Nutrition Facts (per serving):

- Calories: 300
- Carbs: 15g
- Protein: 25g
- Fat: 15g

60. Veggie Bread

Prep.Time: 15 min

Cook Time: 50 min

Serving: 12

Beverage pairing: Herbal Tea

Ingredients:

- 2 cups almond flour
- 1/4 cup flaxseed meal
- 1/4 cup psyllium husk powder
- 1 tablespoon baking powder
- 1/2 teaspoon salt
- 4 large eggs
- 1/4 cup olive oil
- 1/2 cup unsweetened almond milk
- 1 cup grated zucchini
- 1/2 cup grated carrot
- 1/4 cup chopped spinach
- 2 tablespoons chopped fresh parsley
- 1 tablespoon chopped fresh chives

Preparation:

1. Preheat your oven to 350°F (175°C). Grease a loaf pan or line it with parchment paper.
2. In a large bowl, whisk together almond flour, flaxseed meal, psyllium husk powder, baking powder, and salt.
3. In a separate bowl, beat the eggs. Add olive oil and almond milk, and whisk until well combined.
4. Gradually add the wet ingredients to the dry ingredients, stirring until a thick batter forms.
5. Fold in grated zucchini, grated carrot, chopped spinach, parsley, and chives until evenly distributed throughout the batter.
6. Pour the batter into the prepared loaf pan, spreading it out evenly.
7. Bake in the preheated oven for 50-60 minutes, or until the bread is golden brown on top and a toothpick inserted into the center comes out clean.
8. Remove the bread from the oven and let it cool in the pan for 10 minutes.
9. Carefully transfer the bread to a wire rack to cool completely before slicing.

Nutrition Facts (per serving - 1 slice):

- Calories: 150
- Carbohydrates: 7g
- Protein: 6g
- Fat: 12g

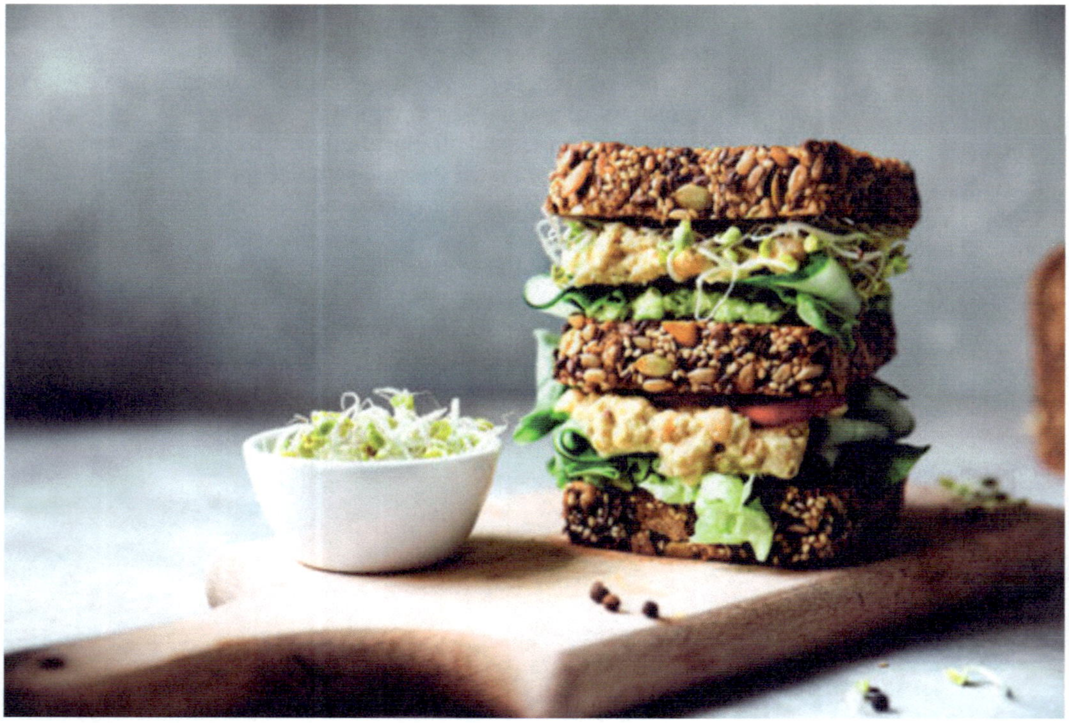

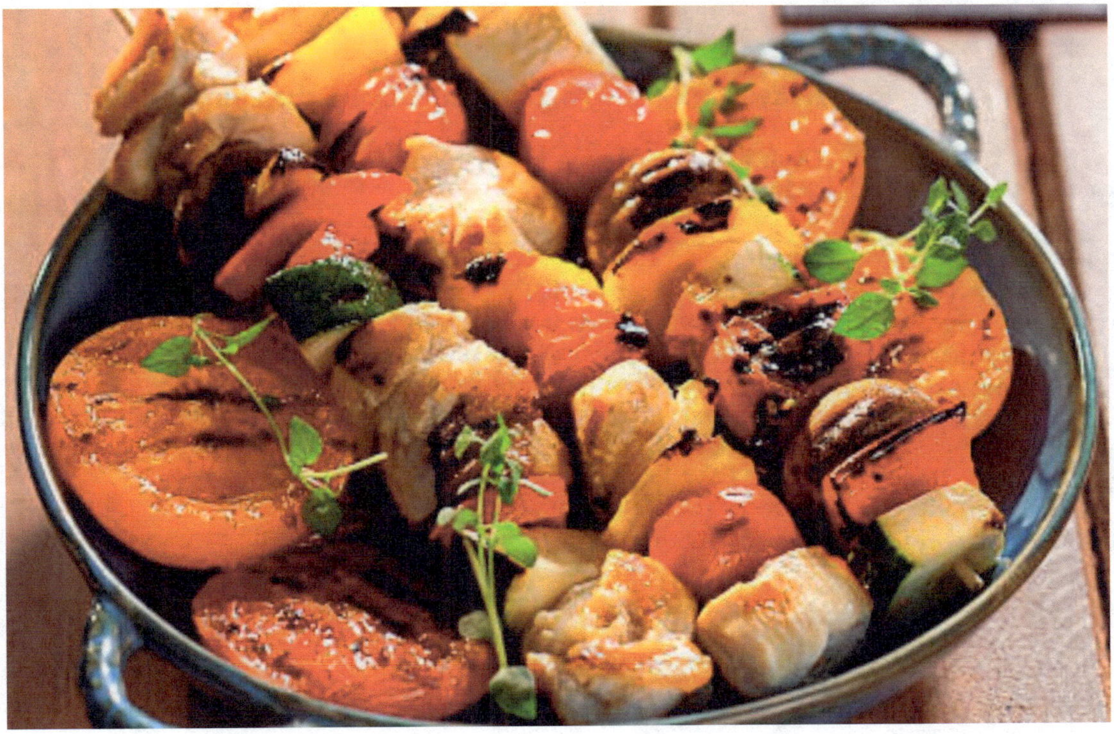

63. Grilled Chicken and Vegetable Kebabs with Herb Marinade

Prep.Time: 20 min

Cook Time: 12 min

Serving: 4

Beverage pairing: Herbal Tea

Ingredients:

- 1 pound boneless, skinless chicken breasts, cut into cubes
- 2 bell peppers (assorted colors), cut into chunks
- 1 red onion, cut into chunks
- 1 zucchini, sliced
- 8-10 cherry tomatoes
- Wooden skewers, soaked in water for 30 minutes
- 1/4 cup olive oil
- 2 tablespoons balsamic vinegar
- 2 cloves garlic, minced
- 2 teaspoons dried Italian herbs (basil, oregano, thyme)

Preparation:

1. In a bowl, whisk together olive oil, balsamic vinegar, minced garlic, dried Italian herbs, salt, and pepper to make the marinade.
2. Thread chicken cubes, bell pepper chunks, red onion chunks, zucchini slices, and cherry tomatoes onto the wooden skewers, alternating the ingredients.
3. Place the assembled kebabs in a shallow dish and pour the herb marinade over them, ensuring they are evenly coated.
4. Cover and refrigerate for at least 30 minutes to marinate.
5. Preheat grill to medium-high heat. Grill kebabs for 10-12 minutes, turning occasionally, or until chicken is cooked through and vegetables are tender.
6. Serve hot.

Nutrition Facts (per serving):

- Calories: 250
- Carbs: 10g
- Protein: 25g
- Fat: 15g

64. Baked Cod with Tomato and Olive Tapenade

Prep.Time: 10 min

Cook Time: 20 min

Serving: 4

Beverage pairing: Iced Tea

Ingredients:

- 4 cod fillets
- 1 cup cherry tomatoes, halved
- 1/4 cup pitted Kalamata olives, chopped
- 2 cloves garlic, minced
- 2 tablespoons olive oil
- 1 tablespoon capers, drained
- 1 teaspoon dried oregano
- Salt and pepper to taste
- Lemon wedges for serving
- Chopped fresh parsley for garnish (optional)

Preparation:

1. Preheat oven to 400°F (200°C).
2. Place cod fillets in a baking dish lined with parchment paper.
3. In a bowl, mix together cherry tomatoes, chopped Kalamata olives, minced garlic, olive oil, capers, dried oregano, salt, and pepper.
4. Spoon the tomato and olive tapenade over the cod fillets, spreading it evenly.
5. Bake in the preheated oven for 15-20 minutes, or until cod is opaque and flakes easily with a fork.
6. Serve hot with lemon wedges on the side.
7. Garnish with chopped fresh parsley if desired before serving.

Nutrition Facts (per serving):

- Calories: 200
- Carbs: 5g
- Protein: 25g
- Fat: 10g

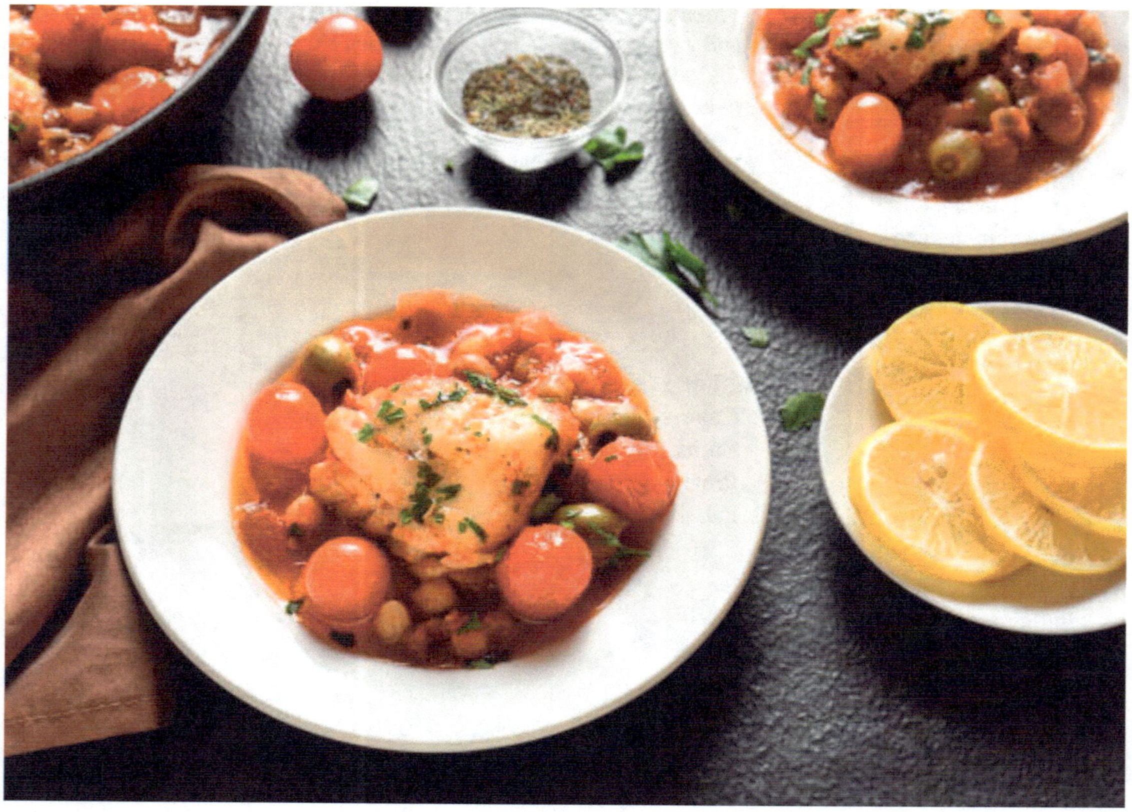

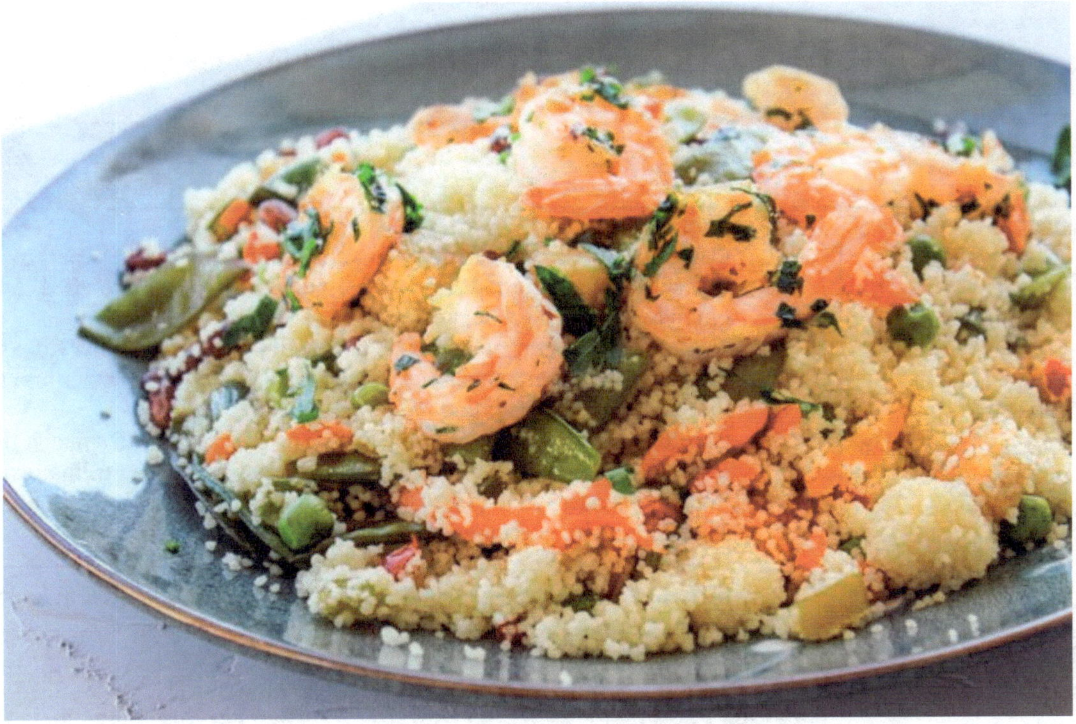

65. Cauliflower and Edamame Fried "Rice" with Shrimp

Prep.Time: 15 min

Cook Time: 15 min

Serving: 4

Beverage pairing: Herbal Tea

Ingredients:

- 1 head cauliflower, grated or processed into rice-like texture
- 1 cup frozen shelled edamame, thawed
- 1 pound large shrimp, peeled and deveined
- 2 tablespoons sesame oil
- 2 cloves garlic, minced
- 2 tablespoons low-sodium soy sauce
- 1 tablespoon rice vinegar
- 2 green onions, sliced
- Salt and pepper to taste
- Optional: Sriracha sauce for serving

Preparation:

1. In a large skillet or wok, heat sesame oil over medium heat. Add minced garlic and cook until fragrant.
2. Add shrimp to the skillet and cook for 2-3 minutes per side, or until pink and cooked through. Remove shrimp from the skillet and set aside.
3. In the same skillet, add grated cauliflower and thawed edamame. Stir-fry for 5-6 minutes, or until cauliflower is tender.
4. Return cooked shrimp to the skillet. Add low-sodium soy sauce and rice vinegar. Stir to combine.
5. Cook for another 2-3 minutes, allowing flavors to meld.
6. Season with salt and pepper to taste. Stir in sliced green onions.
7. Serve hot, optionally drizzled with Sriracha sauce.

Nutrition Facts (per serving):

- Calories: 250
- Carbs: 15g
- Protein: 25g
- Fat: 10g

66. Turkey and Spinach Stuffed Zucchini Blossoms

Prep.Time: 20 min

Cook Time: 20 min

Serving: 6

Beverage pairing: Iced Tea

Ingredients:

- 12 zucchini blossoms
- 1/2 pound ground turkey
- 1 cup chopped spinach
- 1/4 cup diced onion
- 2 cloves garlic, minced
- 1/4 cup grated Parmesan cheese
- 1/4 teaspoon dried oregano
- Salt and pepper to taste
- Olive oil for brushing

Preparation:

1. Carefully rinse zucchini blossoms and gently pat dry with paper towels.
2. In a skillet, cook ground turkey over medium heat until browned. Add diced onion and minced garlic, and cook until softened.
3. Stir in chopped spinach and cook until wilted. Remove skillet from heat.
4. Stir in grated Parmesan cheese, dried oregano, salt, and pepper into the turkey and spinach mixture.
5. Carefully stuff each zucchini blossom with the turkey and spinach filling.
6. Gently twist the ends of the zucchini blossoms to seal the filling inside.
7. Preheat oven to 375°F (190°C). Place stuffed zucchini blossoms on a baking sheet lined with parchment paper.
8. Brush the tops of the stuffed zucchini blossoms with olive oil.
9. Bake in the preheated oven for 15-20 minutes, or until zucchini blossoms are tender and filling is heated through.
10. Serve hot.

Nutrition Facts (per serving, serving size: 2 stuffed zucchini blossoms):

- Calories: 150
- Carbs: 5g
- Protein: 15g
- Fat: 8g

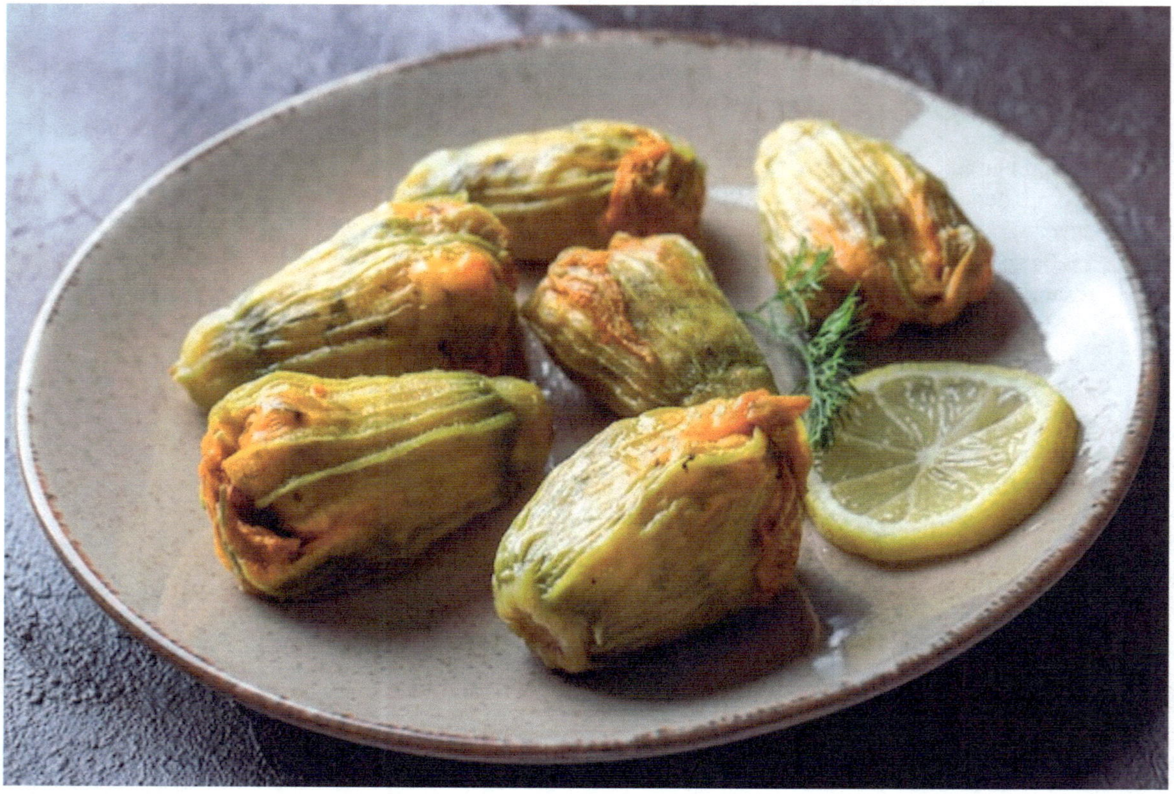

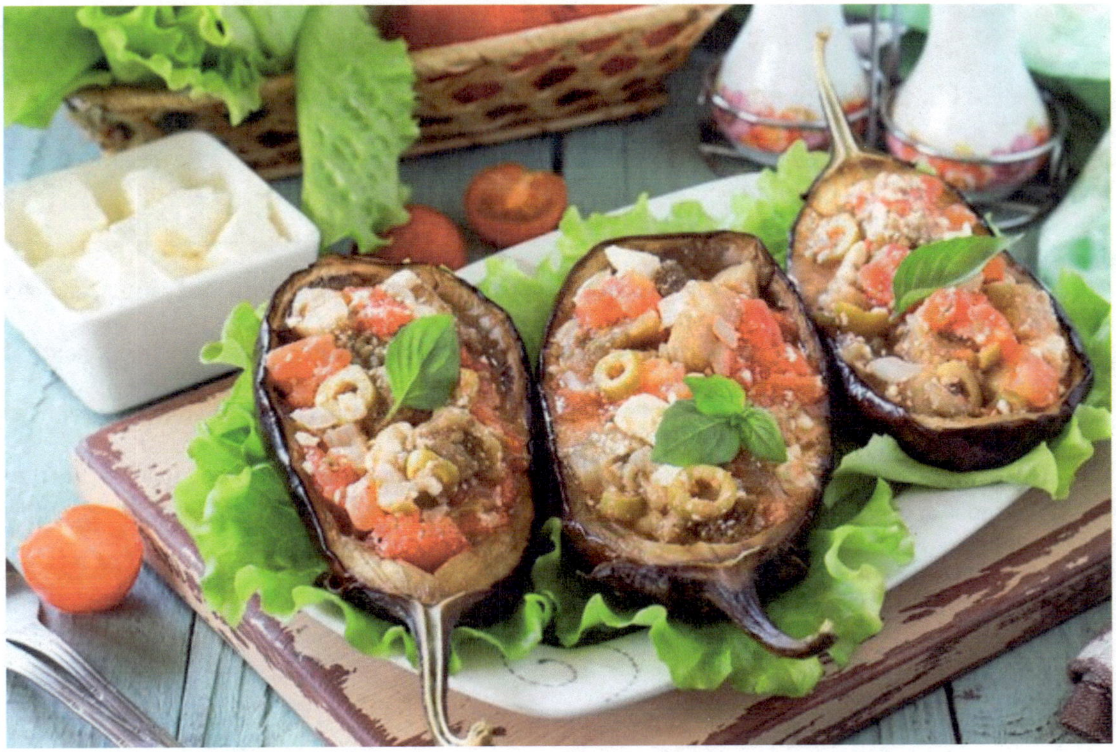

67. Roasted Red Plant and Feta Turkey Meatball Lettuce Cups

Prep.Time: 15 min

Cook Time: 25 min

Serving: 4

Beverage pairing: Herbal Tea

Ingredients:

- 1 pound ground turkey
- 1/4 cup breadcrumbs (whole wheat or low-carb)
- 1/4 cup crumbled feta cheese
- 1/4 cup chopped roasted red plant
- 1/4 cup chopped fresh parsley
- 1 egg
- 2 cloves garlic, minced
- Salt and pepper to taste
- Butter lettuce leaves for serving

Preparation:

1. Preheat oven to 375°F (190°C).
2. In a bowl, mix together ground turkey, breadcrumbs, crumbled feta cheese, chopped roasted red plant, chopped fresh parsley, egg, minced garlic, salt, and pepper until well combined.
3. Shape the turkey mixture into meatballs, about 1 inch in diameter.
4. Place meatballs on a baking sheet lined with parchment paper.
5. Bake in the preheated oven for 20-25 minutes, or until meatballs are cooked through and golden brown.
6. Arrange butter lettuce leaves on a serving platter.
7. Place roasted red plant and feta turkey meatballs on top of the lettuce leaves.
8. Serve hot or at room temperature.

Nutrition Facts (per serving, serving size: 3 meatballs with lettuce):

- Calories: 250
- Carbs: 5g
- Protein: 25g
- Fat: 15g

68. Cabbage and Carrot Slaw with Apple Cider Vinaigrette

Prep.Time: 10 min

Cook Time: 0 min

Serving: 4

Beverage pairing: Iced Tea

Ingredients:

- 4 cups shredded cabbage (green or purple)
- 1 cup shredded carrots
- 1/4 cup chopped fresh parsley
- 2 tablespoons apple cider vinegar
- 1 tablespoon olive oil
- 1 teaspoon honey (or a sugar-free sweetener)
- 1/2 teaspoon Dijon mustard
- Salt and pepper to taste

Preparation:

1. In a large bowl, combine shredded cabbage, shredded carrots, and chopped fresh parsley.
2. In a small bowl, whisk together apple cider vinegar, olive oil, honey, Dijon mustard, salt, and pepper to make the vinaigrette.
3. Pour the vinaigrette over the cabbage and carrot mixture. Toss until evenly coated.
4. Let the slaw sit for at least 10 minutes before serving to allow the flavors to meld.
5. Serve chilled.

Nutrition Facts (per serving):

- Calories: 100
- Carbs: 10g
- Protein: 2g
- Fat: 6g

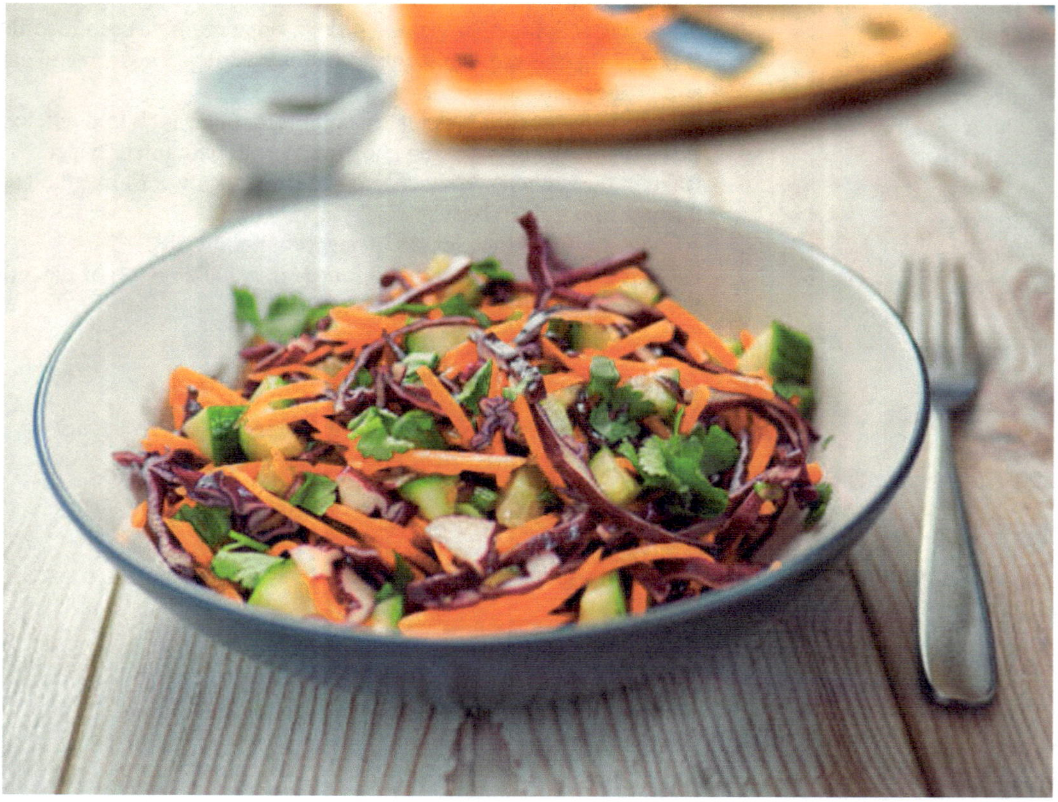

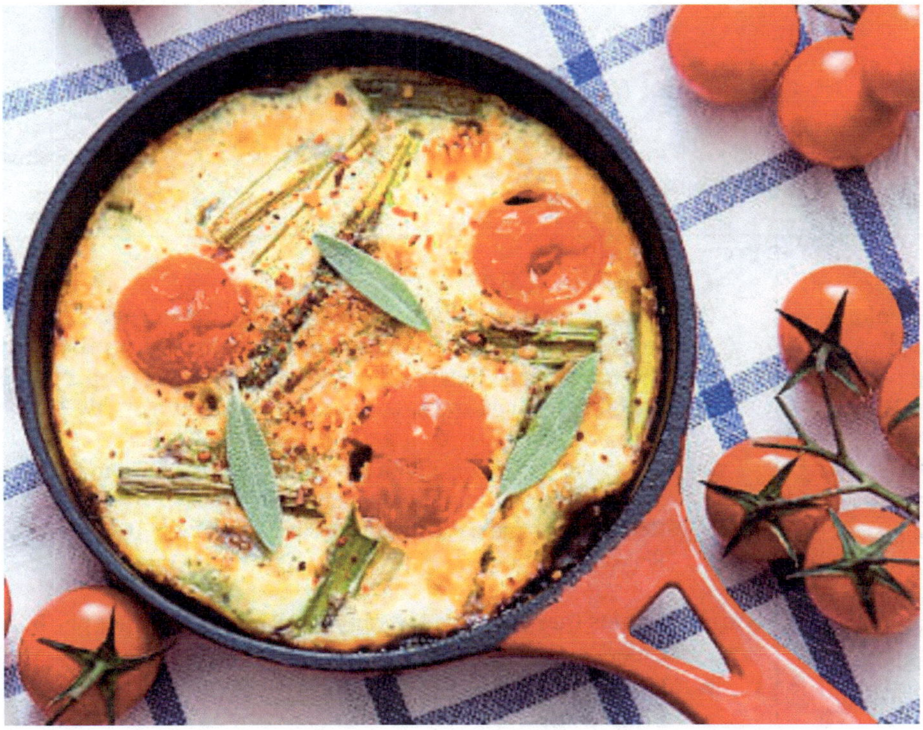

69. Egg White and Vegetable Frittata with Sweet Potato Hash

Prep.Time: 15 min | **Cook Time:** 30 min | **Serving:** 4 | **Beverage pairing:** Herbal Tea

Ingredients:

- 8 egg whites
- 1/2 cup diced bell peppers (assorted colors)
- 1/2 cup diced zucchini
- 1/2 cup diced tomatoes
- 1/4 cup diced onion
- 2 cloves garlic, minced
- 1/4 cup chopped fresh parsley
- Salt and pepper to taste
- 1 tablespoon olive oil
- 2 small sweet potatoes, diced
- 1 tablespoon olive oil
- Salt and pepper to taste

Preparation:

1. Preheat oven to 375°F (190°C).
2. In a bowl, whisk together egg whites, diced bell peppers, diced zucchini, diced tomatoes, minced garlic, chopped fresh parsley, salt, and pepper.
3. Heat olive oil in an oven-safe skillet over medium heat. Add diced onion and cook until softened.
4. Pour the egg white and vegetable mixture into the skillet.
5. Cook for 3-4 minutes, or until the edges begin to set.
6. Transfer the skillet to the preheated oven and bake for 15-20 minutes, or until the frittata is set in the center and lightly golden on top.
7. In the meantime, prepare the sweet potato hash. Heat olive oil in a separate skillet over medium heat. Add diced sweet potatoes and cook until tender, about 10 minutes. Season with salt and pepper to taste.
8. Serve slices of the egg white and vegetable frittata with a side of sweet potato hash.

Nutrition Facts (per serving):

- Calories: 200
- Carbs: 20g
- Protein: 15g
- Fat: 8g

70. Quinoa and Roasted Vegetable Stuffed Bell Peppers

Prep.Time: 20 min

Cook Time: 35 min

Serving: 4

Beverage pairing: Iced Tea

Ingredients:

- 4 bell peppers (assorted colors), halved and seeds removed
- 1 cup cooked quinoa
- 1 cup diced roasted vegetables (e.g., bell peppers, zucchini, eggplant)
- 1/4 cup crumbled feta cheese
- 2 tablespoons chopped fresh parsley
- 1 tablespoon olive oil
- Salt and pepper to taste

Preparation:

1. Preheat oven to 375°F (190°C).
2. Place bell pepper halves in a baking dish, cut side up.
3. In a bowl, combine cooked quinoa, diced roasted vegetables, crumbled feta cheese, chopped fresh parsley, olive oil, salt, and pepper.
4. Spoon the quinoa and roasted vegetable mixture evenly into each bell pepper half.
5. Cover the baking dish with aluminum foil and bake in the preheated oven for 25-30 minutes, or until bell peppers are tender.
6. Remove foil and bake for an additional 5 minutes to lightly brown the tops.
7. Serve hot.

Nutrition Facts (per serving, serving size: 2 stuffed bell pepper halves):

- Calories: 250
- Carbs: 30g
- Protein: 10g
- Fat: 10g

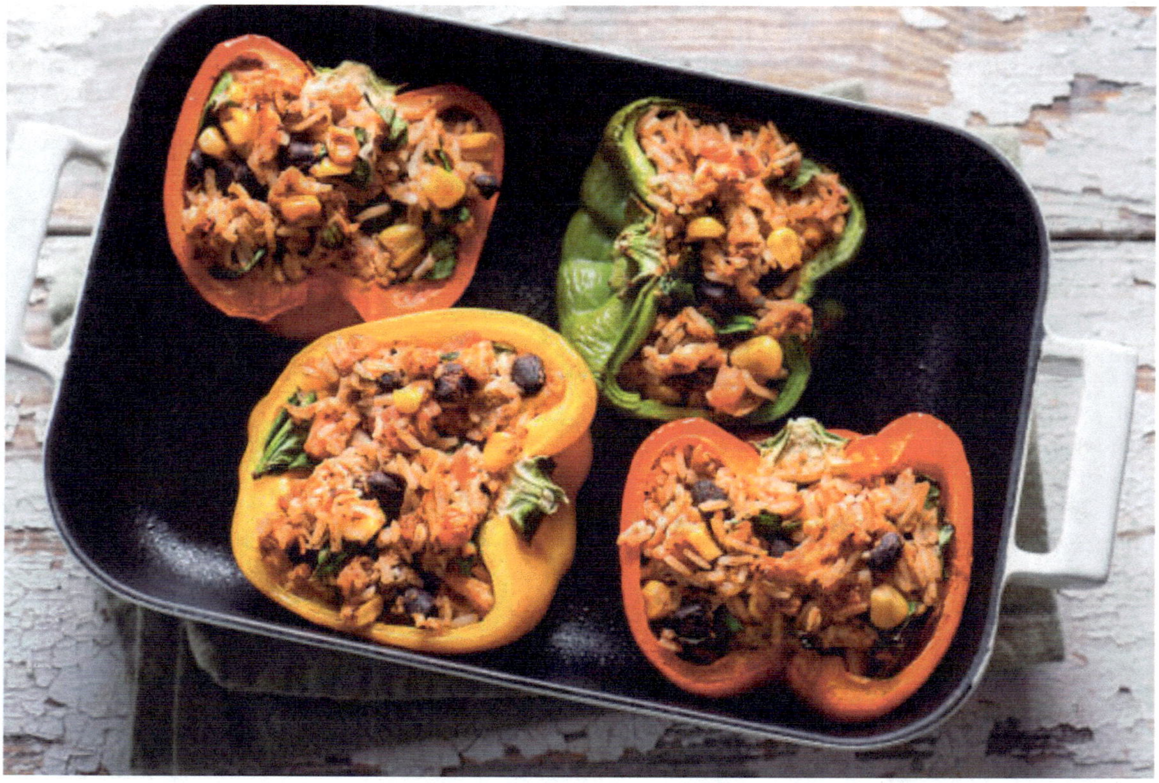

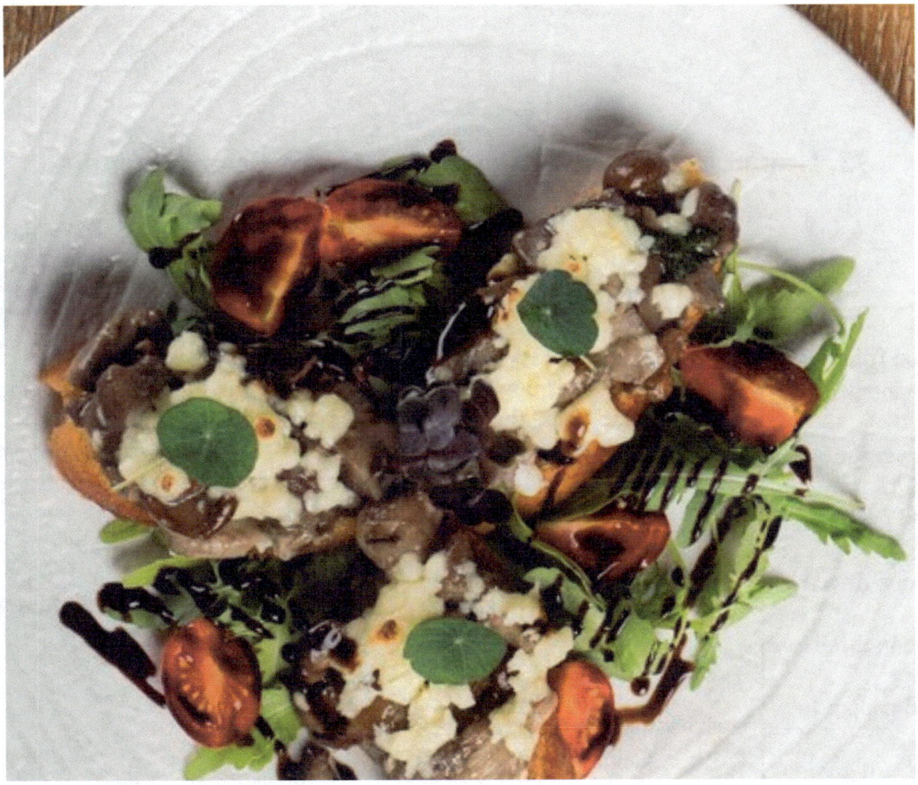

71. Grilled Tofu and Portobello Mushroom Salad with Balsamic Reduction

Prep.Time: 15 min

Cook Time: 10 min

Serving: 4

Beverage pairing: Herbal Tea

Ingredients:

- 1 block extra-firm tofu, pressed and sliced
- 2 large Portobello mushrooms, stems removed and sliced
- 4 cups mixed salad greens
- 1 cup cherry tomatoes, halved
- 1/4 cup balsamic vinegar
- 1 tablespoon olive oil
- 1 teaspoon honey (or a sugar-free sweetener)
- Salt and pepper to taste
- Fresh basil leaves for garnish (optional)

Preparation:

1. Preheat grill to medium-high heat.
2. In a small saucepan, combine balsamic vinegar and honey. Bring to a simmer over medium heat and cook until the mixture is reduced by half, stirring occasionally. Set aside.
3. Lightly brush sliced tofu and Portobello mushrooms with olive oil. Season with salt and pepper.
4. Grill tofu slices and Portobello mushroom slices for 4-5 minutes per side, or until grill marks appear and they are heated through.
5. In a large bowl, toss mixed salad greens and cherry tomatoes with olive oil.
6. Arrange grilled tofu slices and Portobello mushroom slices on top of the salad.
7. Drizzle with balsamic reduction.
8. Garnish with fresh basil leaves if desired before serving.

Nutrition Facts (per serving):

- Calories: 250
- Carbs: 15g
- Protein: 15g
- Fat: 15g

72. Lemon Herb Baked Salmon with Green Bean Almondine

Prep.Time: 10 min

Cook Time: 20 min

Serving: 4

Beverage pairing: Iced Tea

Ingredients:

- 4 salmon fillets
- 2 tablespoons olive oil
- 2 cloves garlic, minced
- Zest and juice of 1 lemon
- 1 teaspoon dried thyme
- 1 teaspoon dried rosemary
- Salt and pepper to taste
- 2 cups fresh green beans, trimmed
- 1/4 cup sliced almonds

Preparation:

1. Preheat oven to 375°F (190°C).
2. In a small bowl, whisk together olive oil, minced garlic, lemon zest, lemon juice, dried thyme, dried rosemary, salt, and pepper.
3. Place salmon fillets in a baking dish lined with parchment paper.
4. Pour the lemon herb marinade over the salmon fillets, ensuring they are evenly coated.
5. Arrange green beans around the salmon fillets in the baking dish.
6. Sprinkle sliced almonds over the green beans.
7. Bake in the preheated oven for 15-20 minutes, or until salmon is cooked through and flakes easily with a fork.
8. Serve hot.

Nutrition Facts (per serving):

- Calories: 300
- Carbs: 10g
- Protein: 25g
- Fat: 20g

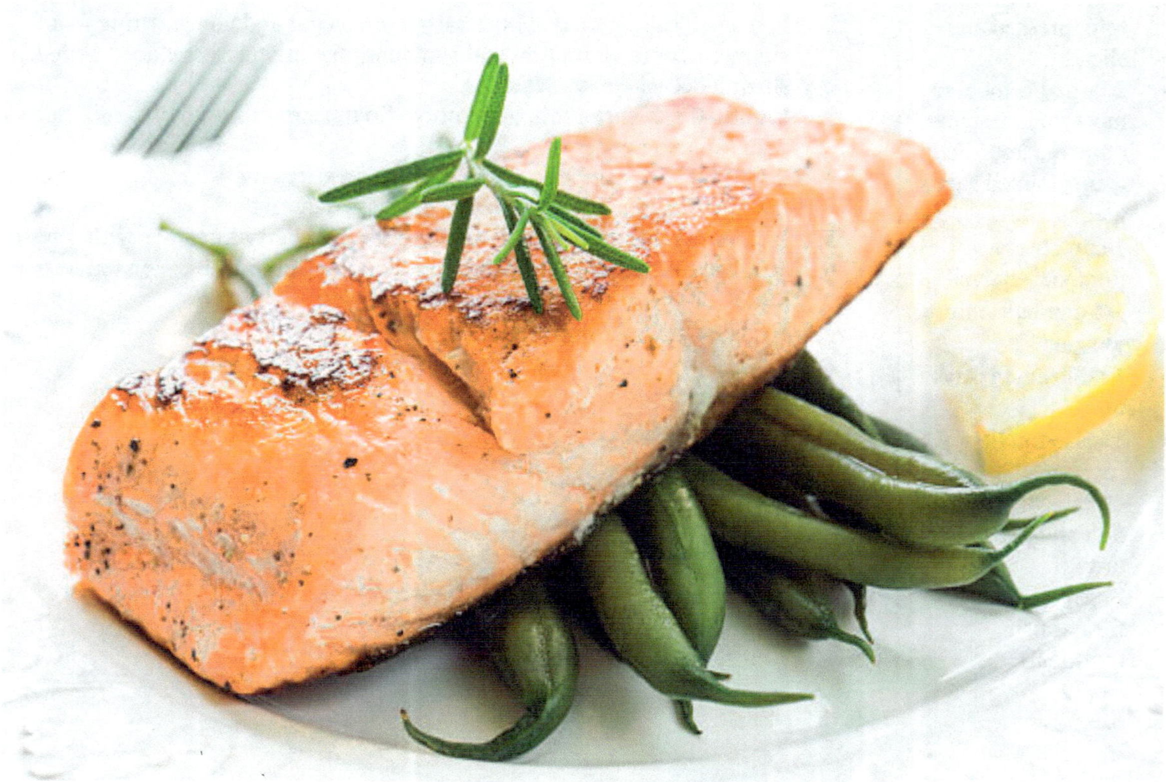

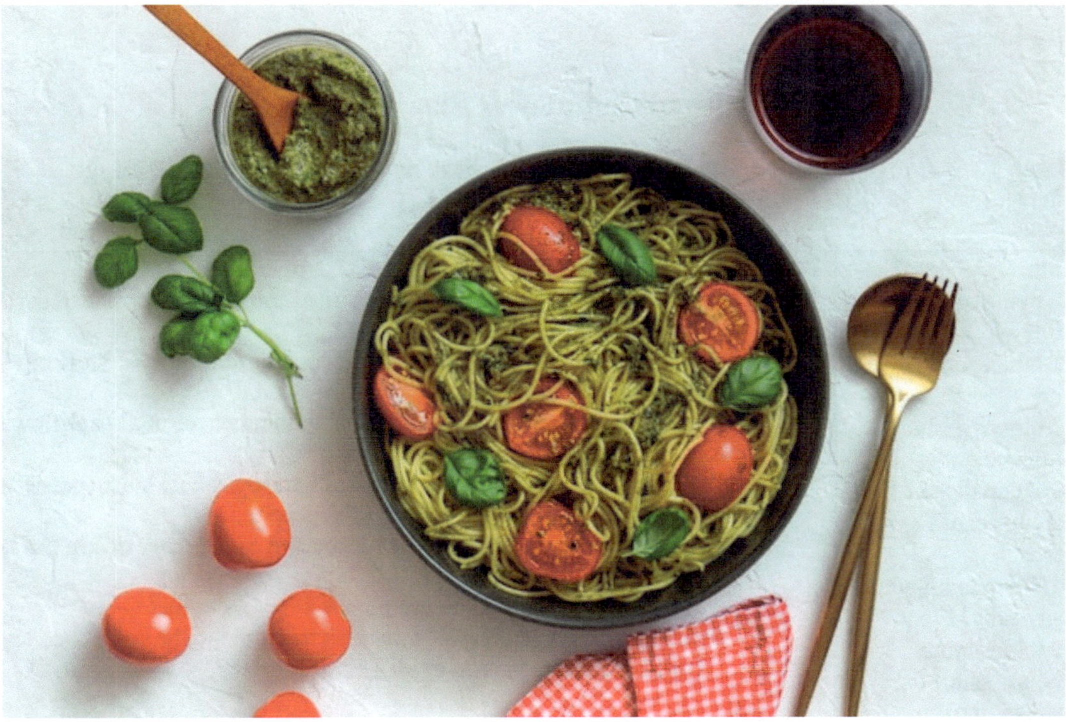

73. Zucchini Ribbon and Tomato Salad with Basil Pesto

Prep.Time: 15 min

Cook Time: 0 min

Serving: 4

Beverage pairing: Herbal Tea

Ingredients:

- 3 medium zucchinis
- 1 cup cherry tomatoes, halved
- 1/4 cup prepared basil pesto (store-bought or homemade)
- 2 tablespoons pine nuts, toasted
- Salt and pepper to taste
- Fresh basil leaves for garnish (optional)

Preparation:

1. Use a vegetable peeler to create long ribbons from the zucchinis. Place the ribbons in a large bowl.
2. Add halved cherry tomatoes to the bowl with the zucchini ribbons.
3. In a small bowl, mix together basil pesto, toasted pine nuts, salt, and pepper.
4. Pour the basil pesto mixture over the zucchini ribbons and cherry tomatoes. Toss until evenly coated.
5. Garnish with fresh basil leaves if desired before serving.

Nutrition Facts (per serving):

- Calories: 200
- Carbs: 10g
- Protein: 5g
- Fat: 15g

74. Turkey and Cauliflower Rice Lettuce Wraps

Prep.Time: 15 min

Cook Time: 15 min

Serving: 4

Beverage pairing: Herbal Tea

Ingredients:

- 1 pound ground turkey
- 1 tablespoon olive oil
- 2 cloves garlic, minced
- 1/2 cup diced onion
- 2 cups cauliflower rice
- 1/4 cup low-sodium soy sauce
- 2 tablespoons hoisin sauce (or a sugar-free alternative)
- 1 teaspoon sesame oil
- Butter lettuce leaves for serving
- Sliced green onions for garnish

Preparation:

1. In a large skillet, heat olive oil over medium heat. Add minced garlic and diced onion, and sauté until softened.
2. Add ground turkey to the skillet and cook until browned, breaking it into small pieces as it cooks.
3. Stir in cauliflower rice and cook for 5-6 minutes, or until cauliflower is tender.
4. In a small bowl, mix together low-sodium soy sauce, hoisin sauce, sesame oil, sriracha sauce (if using), salt, and pepper.
5. Pour the sauce mixture over the turkey and cauliflower rice in the skillet. Stir to combine.
6. Cook for another 2-3 minutes, allowing flavors to meld.
7. Spoon the turkey and cauliflower rice mixture into butter lettuce leaves.
8. Garnish with sliced green onions before serving.

Nutrition Facts (per serving):

- Calories: 250
- Carbs: 10g
- Protein: 25g
- Fat: 15g

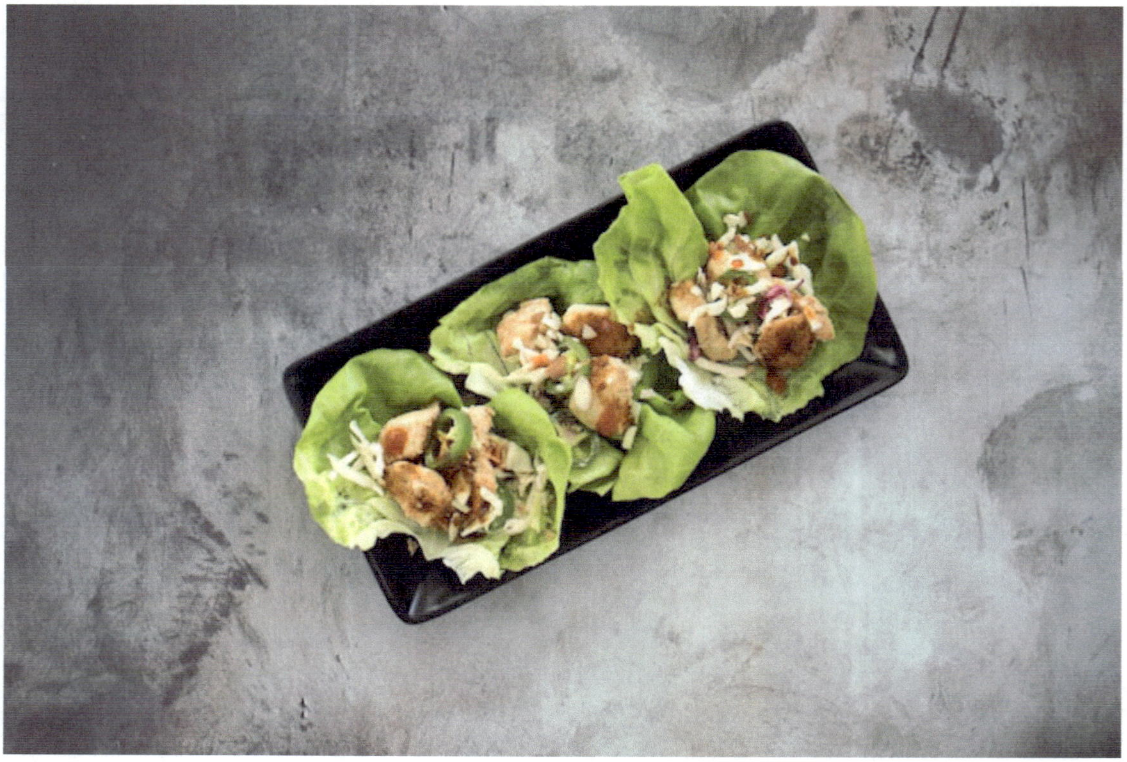

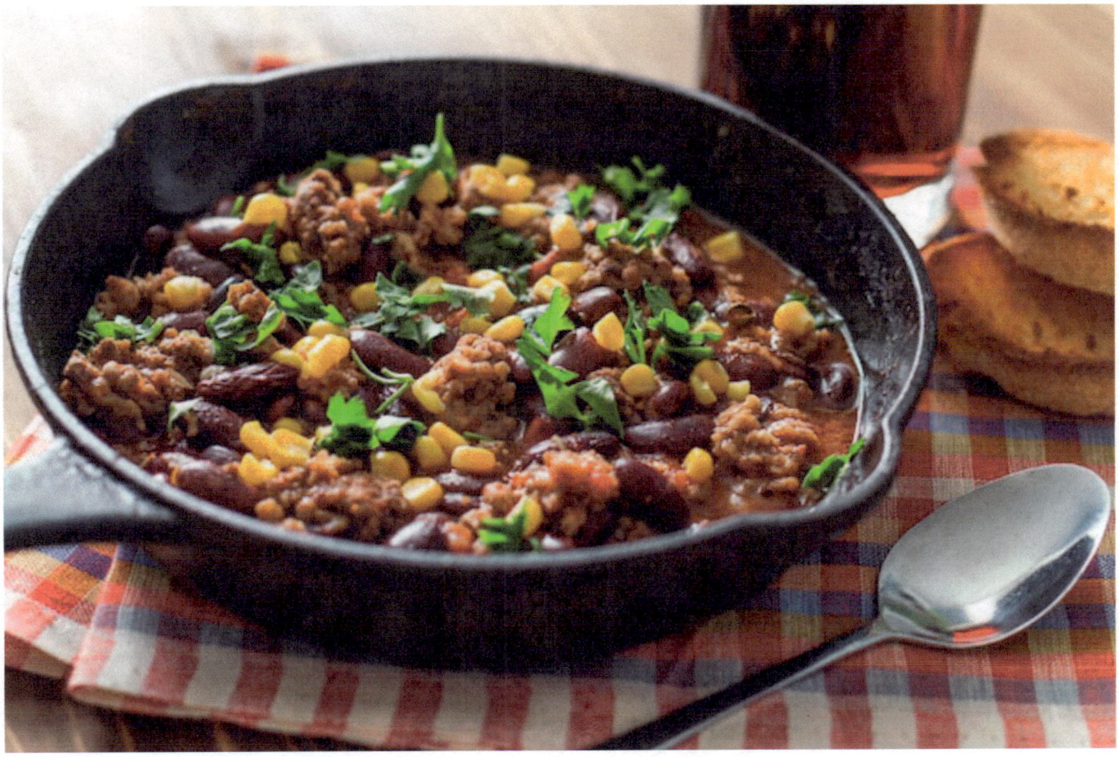

75. Eggplant and Chickpea Tagine with Quinoa

Prep.Time: 15 min

Cook Time: 30 min

Serving: 4

Beverage pairing: Herbal Tea

Ingredients:

- 1 large eggplant, diced
- 1 can (15 oz) chickpeas, drained and rinsed
- 1 onion, diced
- 2 cloves garlic, minced
- 1 can (15 oz) diced tomatoes
- 1 tablespoon tomato paste
- 1 teaspoon ground cumin
- 1 teaspoon ground coriander
- 1/2 teaspoon smoked paprika
- 1/4 teaspoon cinnamon
- Salt and pepper to taste
- 2 cups cooked quinoa

Preparation:

1. In a large pot or Dutch oven, heat olive oil over medium heat. Add diced onion and minced garlic, and sauté until softened.
2. Add diced eggplant to the pot and cook until lightly browned.
3. Stir in drained and rinsed chickpeas, diced tomatoes, tomato paste, ground cumin, ground coriander, smoked paprika, cinnamon, salt, and pepper.
4. Bring the mixture to a simmer, then reduce heat to low. Cover and cook for 20-25 minutes, stirring occasionally, or until eggplant is tender.
5. Serve the eggplant and chickpea tagine over cooked quinoa.
6. Garnish with chopped fresh cilantro if desired before serving.

Nutrition Facts (per serving):

- Calories: 300
- Carbs: 45g
- Protein: 10g
- Fat: 8g

76. Shrimp and Avocado Cucumber Roll-Ups

Prep.Time: 15 min

Cook Time: 0 min

Serving: 4

Beverage pairing: Herbal Tea

Ingredients:

- 1 large cucumber
- 1 avocado, mashed
- 8 large cooked shrimp, peeled and deveined
- 1 tablespoon chopped fresh cilantro
- 1 tablespoon lime juice
- Salt and pepper to taste

Preparation:

1. Using a vegetable peeler, slice the cucumber lengthwise into thin strips.
2. In a small bowl, mix together mashed avocado, chopped cilantro, lime juice, salt, and pepper.
3. Lay out cucumber slices and spread a thin layer of avocado mixture on each slice.
4. Place a cooked shrimp at one end of each cucumber slice.
5. Roll up the cucumber slices with the avocado mixture and shrimp inside.
6. Secure with toothpicks if necessary.
7. Serve chilled.

Nutrition Facts (per serving, serving size: 2 roll-ups):

- Calories: 150
- Carbs: 7g
- Protein: 8g
- Fat: 10g

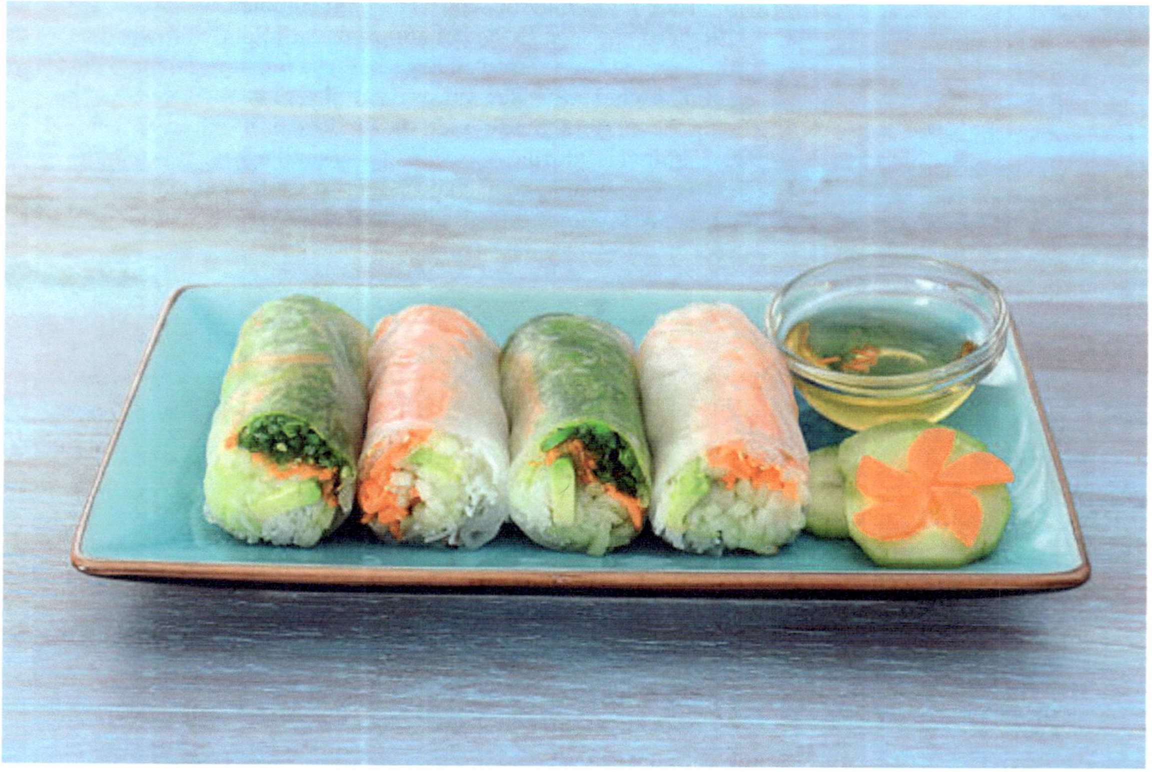

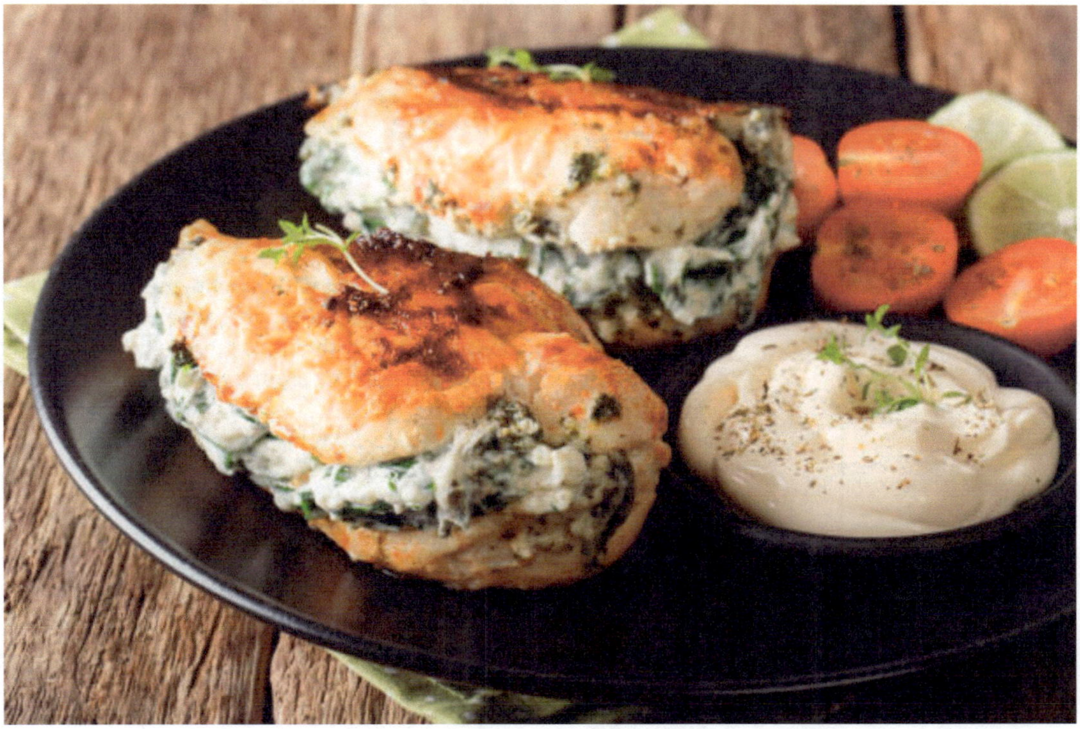

77. Spinach and Feta Stuffed Chicken Thighs

Prep.Time: 15 min

Cook Time: 30 min

Serving: 4

Beverage pairing: Herbal Tea

Ingredients:

- 4 boneless, skinless chicken thighs
- 2 cups fresh spinach leaves
- 1/4 cup crumbled feta cheese
- 2 cloves garlic, minced
- Salt and pepper to taste
- Olive oil for brushing

Preparation:

1. Preheat oven to 375°F (190°C).
2. Place chicken thighs on a cutting board and flatten them with a meat mallet.
3. In a bowl, combine fresh spinach leaves, crumbled feta cheese, minced garlic, salt, and pepper.
4. Spoon the spinach and feta mixture onto each chicken thigh.
5. Roll up the chicken thighs and secure with toothpicks if necessary.
6. Place the stuffed chicken thighs in a baking dish lined with parchment paper.
7. Brush the tops of the stuffed chicken thighs with olive oil.
8. Bake in the preheated oven for 25-30 minutes, or until chicken is cooked through and juices run clear.
9. Serve hot.

Nutrition Facts (per serving):

- Calories: 250
- Carbs: 2g
- Protein: 25g
- Fat: 15g

78. Baked Cod with Lemon Dill Zucchini Noodles

Prep.Time: 15 min

Cook Time: 20 min

Serving: 4

Beverage pairing: Herbal Tea

Ingredients:

- 4 cod fillets
- 2 medium zucchinis, spiralized into noodles
- 2 tablespoons olive oil
- 2 cloves garlic, minced
- Zest and juice of 1 lemon
- 1 tablespoon chopped fresh dill
- Salt and pepper to taste

Preparation:

1. Preheat oven to 375°F (190°C).
2. Place cod fillets in a baking dish lined with parchment paper.
3. In a bowl, toss spiralized zucchini noodles with olive oil, minced garlic, lemon zest, lemon juice, chopped fresh dill, salt, and pepper.
4. Arrange the seasoned zucchini noodles around the cod fillets in the baking dish.
5. Bake in the preheated oven for 15-20 minutes, or until cod is cooked through and flakes easily with a fork.
6. Serve hot.

Nutrition Facts (per serving):

- Calories: 200
- Carbs: 5g
- Protein: 25g
- Fat: 10g

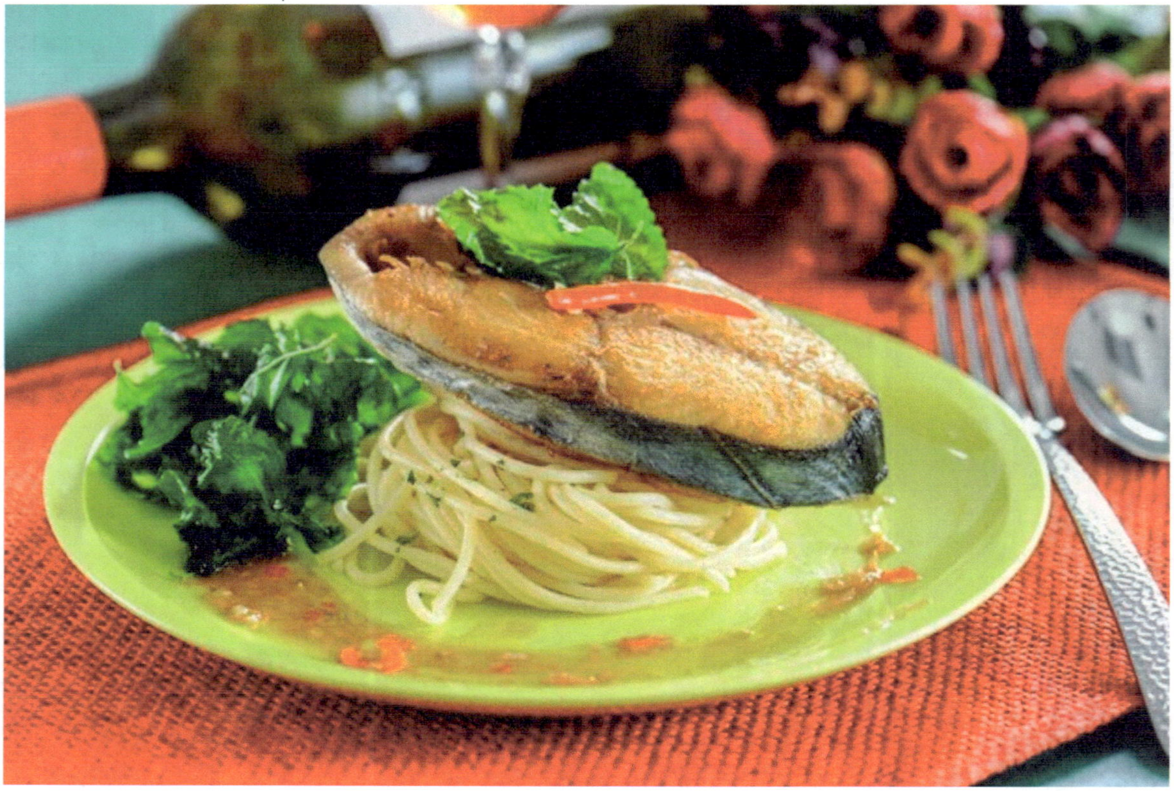

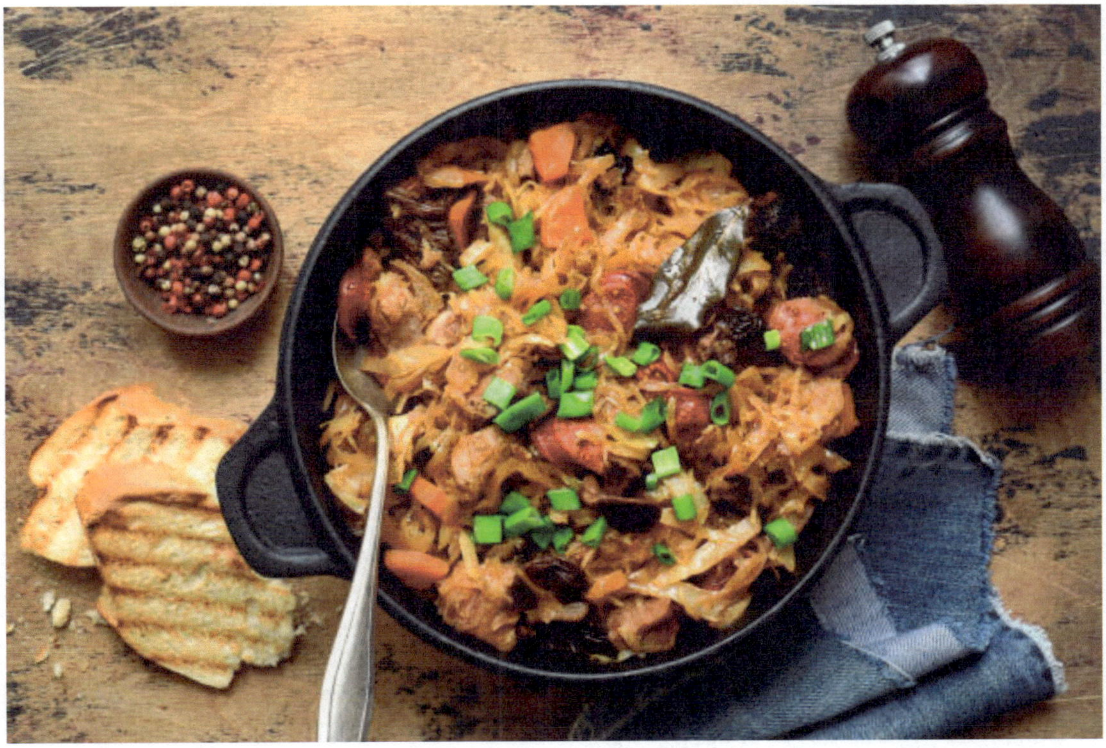

79. Cabbage and Turkey Sausage Stir-Fry with Teriyaki Glaze

Prep.Time: 15 min

Cook Time: 15 min

Serving: 4

Beverage pairing: Herbal Tea

Ingredients:

- 1 pound turkey sausage, sliced
- 4 cups shredded cabbage (green or purple)
- 1 cup shredded carrots
- 1 bell pepper, sliced
- 1/4 cup low-sodium teriyaki sauce
- 2 tablespoons olive oil
- 2 cloves garlic, minced
- Salt and pepper to taste
- Sesame seeds for garnish (optional)
- Sliced green onions for garnish (optional)

Preparation:

1. In a large skillet or wok, heat olive oil over medium heat. Add minced garlic and cook until fragrant.
2. Add sliced turkey sausage to the skillet and cook until browned.
3. Add shredded cabbage, shredded carrots, and sliced bell pepper to the skillet. Stir-fry for 5-6 minutes, or until vegetables are tender-crisp.
4. Pour low-sodium teriyaki sauce over the turkey sausage and vegetables in the skillet. Stir to coat evenly.
5. Cook for another 2-3 minutes, allowing flavors to meld.
6. Season with salt and pepper to taste.
7. Garnish with sesame seeds and sliced green onions if desired before serving.

Nutrition Facts (per serving):

- Calories: 300
- Carbs: 15g
- Protein: 20g
- Fat: 15g

80. Cauliflower and Chickpea Tabbouleh with Grilled Chicken

Prep.Time: 20 min

Cook Time: 0 min

Serving: 4

Beverage pairing: Herbal Tea

Ingredients:

- 1 head cauliflower, grated or processed into rice-like texture
- 1 can (15 oz) chickpeas, drained and rinsed
- 1 cucumber, diced
- 1 tomato, diced
- 1/4 cup chopped fresh parsley
- 1/4 cup chopped fresh mint
- 1/4 cup olive oil
- 2 tablespoons lemon juice
- 2 cloves garlic, minced
- Salt and pepper to taste
- 4 grilled chicken breasts

Preparation:

1. In a large bowl, combine grated cauliflower, drained and rinsed chickpeas, diced cucumber, diced tomato, chopped fresh parsley, and chopped fresh mint.
2. In a small bowl, whisk together olive oil, lemon juice, minced garlic, salt, and pepper to make the dressing.
3. Pour the dressing over the cauliflower and chickpea mixture. Toss until evenly coated.
4. Let the tabbouleh sit for at least 10 minutes before serving to allow the flavors to meld.
5. Serve grilled chicken breasts with cauliflower and chickpea tabbouleh on the side.

Nutrition Facts (per serving):

- Calories: 300
- Carbs: 15g
- Protein: 25g
- Fat: 15g

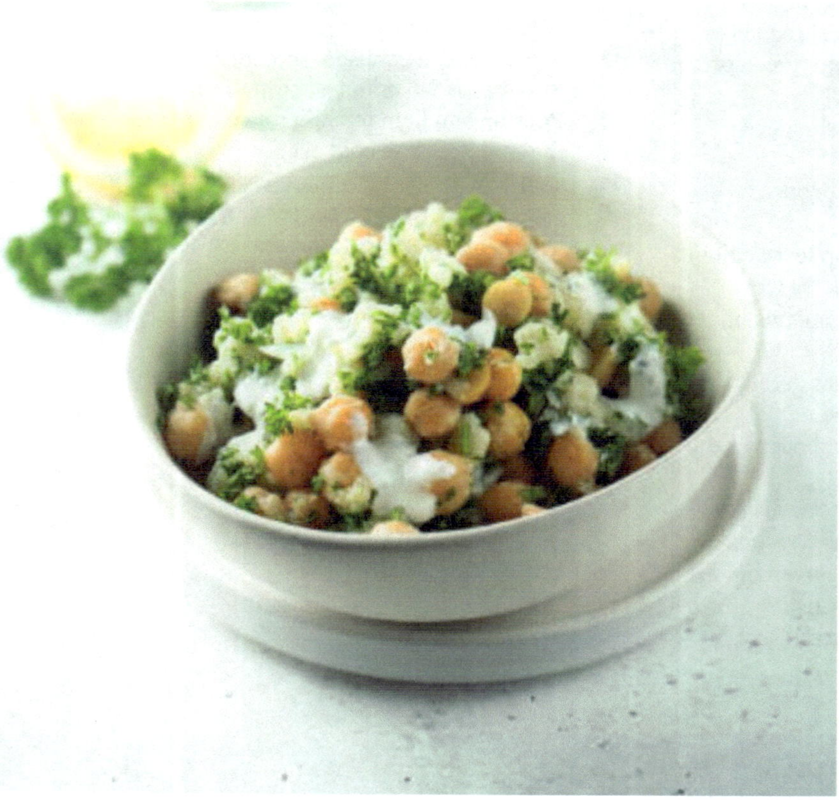

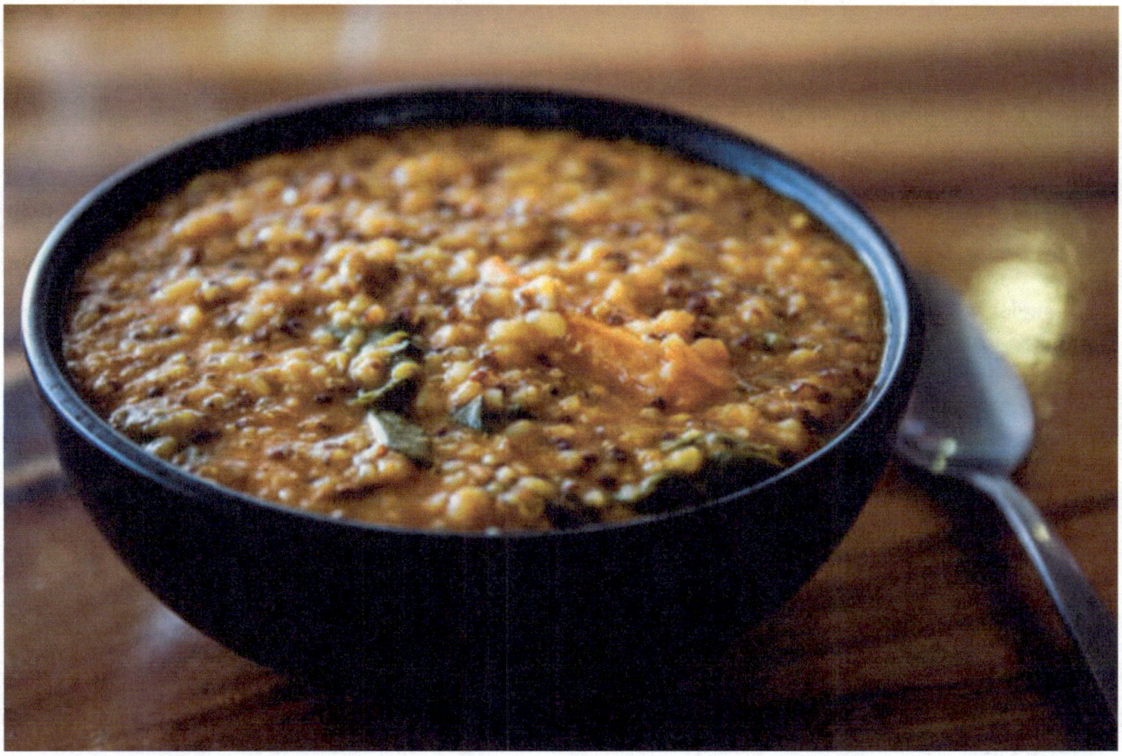

81. Quinoa and Lentil Soup with Spinach

Prep.Time: 10 min

Cook Time: 30 min

Serving: 6

Beverage pairing: Lemonade

Ingredients:

- 1 cup quinoa, rinsed
- 1/2 cup green or brown lentils, rinsed
- 1 onion, chopped
- 2 carrots, diced
- 2 celery stalks, diced
- 3 cloves garlic, minced
- 6 cups vegetable broth
- 2 cups fresh spinach leaves
- 1 teaspoon dried thyme
- 1 teaspoon dried oregano
- Olive oil for cooking

Preparation:

1. In a large pot, heat olive oil over medium heat. Add chopped onion, diced carrots, and diced celery. Cook until vegetables are softened, about 5 minutes.
2. Add minced garlic to the pot and cook for another minute until fragrant.
3. Pour in vegetable broth, rinsed quinoa, and rinsed lentils. Add dried thyme and dried oregano. Season with salt and pepper to taste.
4. Bring the soup to a boil, then reduce the heat to low. Simmer uncovered for about 20-25 minutes, or until the quinoa and lentils are cooked through and tender.
5. Stir in fresh spinach leaves and cook for an additional 2-3 minutes until wilted.
6. Taste and adjust seasoning if needed. Serve hot.

Nutrition Facts (per serving):

- Calories: 250
- Carbohydrates: 45g
- Protein: 12g
- Fat: 3g

82. Grilled Chicken and Asparagus Caesar Salad

Prep.Time: 15 min

Cook Time: 15 min

Serving: 2

Beverage pairing: Lemonade

Ingredients:

- 2 boneless, skinless chicken breasts
- 1 bunch asparagus, ends trimmed
- 1 tablespoon olive oil
- Salt and pepper to taste
- 1 head romaine lettuce, chopped
- 1/4 cup grated Parmesan cheese
- Caesar dressing (store-bought or homemade)
- Croutons (optional)

Preparation:

1. Preheat grill to medium-high heat.
2. Brush chicken breasts and asparagus with olive oil. Season with salt and pepper.
3. Grill chicken breasts for 6-8 minutes per side, or until cooked through and no longer pink in the center. Grill asparagus for 3-4 minutes, or until tender and lightly charred.
4. Remove chicken and asparagus from the grill and let rest for a few minutes. Slice the chicken breasts into strips.
5. In a large bowl, combine chopped romaine lettuce, grilled asparagus, sliced grilled chicken, and grated Parmesan cheese.
6. Drizzle Caesar dressing over the salad and toss to coat evenly.
7. Serve immediately, garnished with croutons if desired.

Nutrition Facts (per serving):

- Calories: 300
- Carbohydrates: 9g
- Protein: 30g
- Fat: 15g

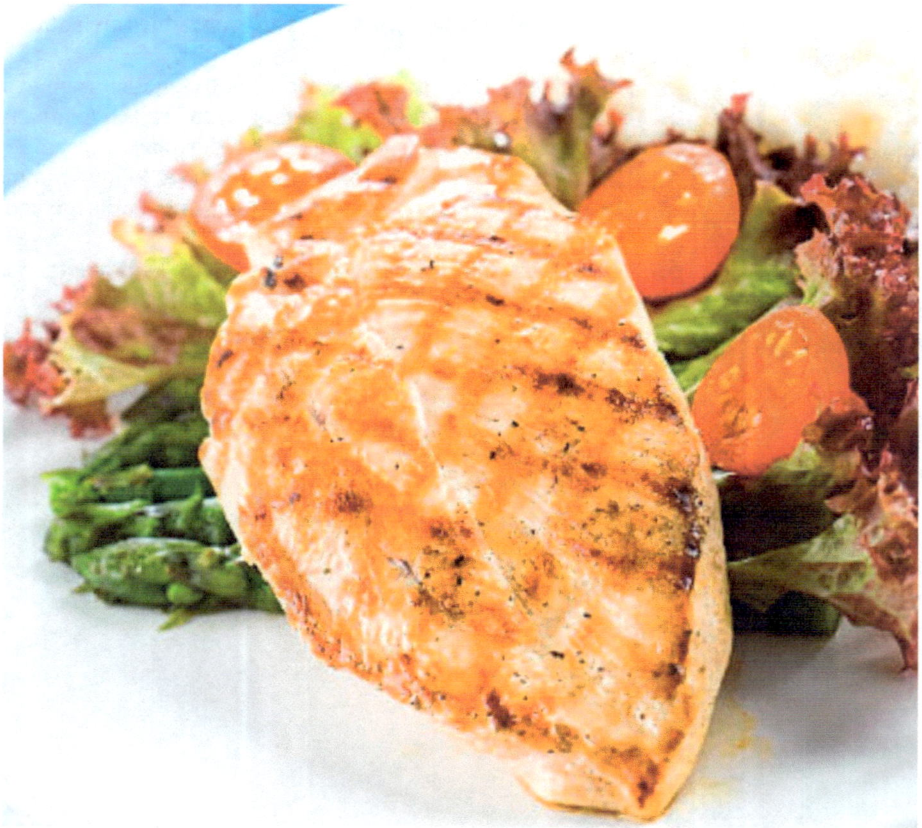

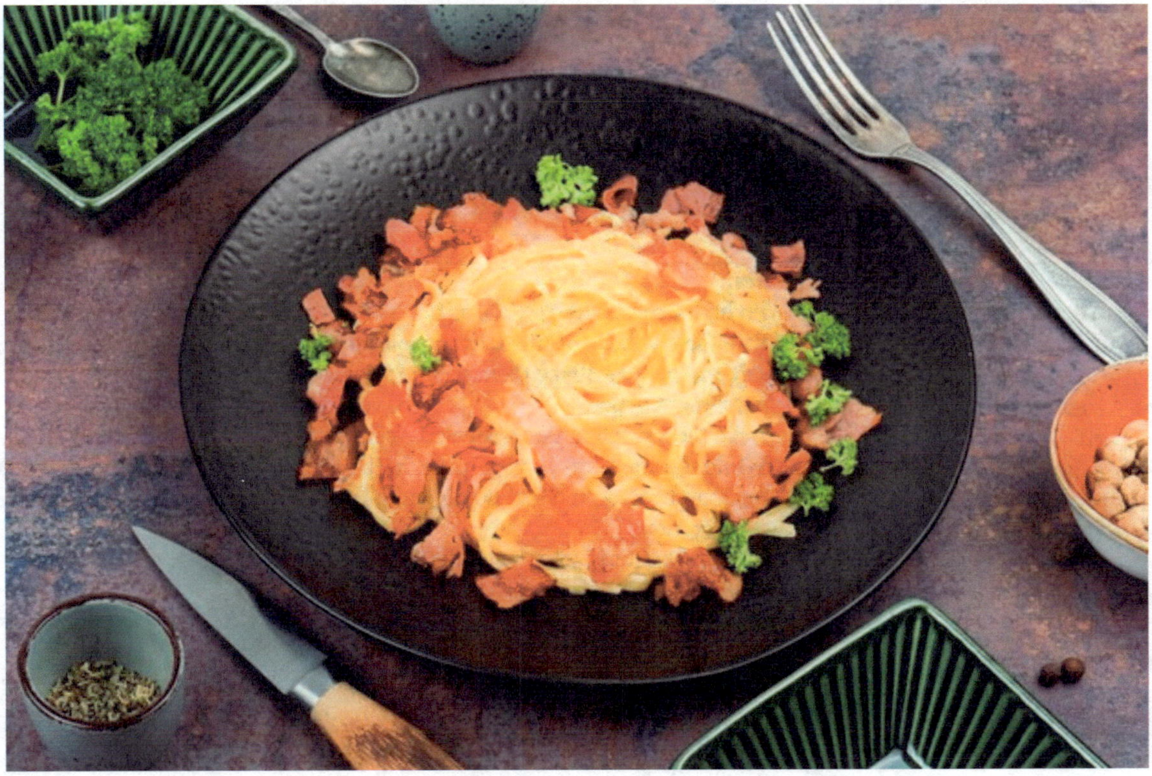

83. Zoodle (Zucchini Noodle) Carbonara with Turkey Bacon

Prep.Time: 15 min

Cook Time: 10 min

Serving: 4

Beverage pairing: Mint water

Ingredients:

- 4 medium zucchini, spiralized into noodles
- 4 slices turkey bacon, diced
- 2 cloves garlic, minced
- 2 eggs
- 1/2 cup grated Parmesan cheese
- Salt and pepper to taste
- Chopped fresh parsley for garnish

Preparation:

1. In a large skillet, cook diced turkey bacon over medium heat until crispy. Remove bacon from the skillet and set aside.
2. In the same skillet with the bacon drippings, add minced garlic and cook until fragrant.
3. Add spiralized zucchini noodles to the skillet and toss to coat in the bacon drippings. Cook for 2-3 minutes until slightly softened but still al dente.
4. In a small bowl, whisk together eggs and grated Parmesan cheese.
5. Remove the skillet from heat and quickly pour the egg and cheese mixture over the zucchini noodles. Toss continuously to coat the noodles evenly and prevent the eggs from scrambling.
6. Add cooked turkey bacon back to the skillet. Season with salt and pepper to taste.
7. Garnish with chopped fresh parsley before serving.

Nutrition Facts (per serving):

- Calories: 200
- Carbohydrates: 10g
- Protein: 15g
- Fat: 12g

84. Turkey and Spinach Stuffed Delicata Squash

Prep.Time: 15 min

Cook Time: 40 min

Serving: 4

Beverage pairing: Lemonade

Ingredients:

- 2 delicata squash, halved and seeds removed
- 1 tablespoon olive oil
- Salt and pepper to taste
- 1/2 lb ground turkey
- 1 small onion, diced
- 2 cloves garlic, minced
- 2 cups fresh spinach leaves
- 1/4 teaspoon dried thyme
- 1/4 teaspoon dried sage
- 1/4 cup grated Parmesan cheese (optional)

Preparation:

1. Preheat oven to 400°F (200°C).
2. Rub the cut sides of the delicata squash halves with olive oil and season with salt and pepper. Place them cut-side down on a baking sheet lined with parchment paper.
3. Bake the squash in the preheated oven for 25-30 minutes, or until tender.
4. While the squash is baking, prepare the filling. In a skillet, heat olive oil over medium heat. Add diced onion and minced garlic, and cook until softened and fragrant.
5. Add ground turkey to the skillet and cook until browned and cooked through.
6. Stir in fresh spinach leaves and cook until wilted. Season with dried thyme, dried sage, salt, and pepper.
7. Once the squash halves are cooked, remove them from the oven and flip them over. Fill each squash half with the turkey and spinach mixture.
8. If desired, sprinkle grated Parmesan cheese over the stuffed squash.
9. Return the stuffed squash to the oven and bake for an additional 10 minutes, or until the cheese is melted and golden brown.
10. Serve hot as a nutritious and satisfying meal.

Nutrition Facts (per serving):

- Calories: 250
- Carbohydrates: 30g
- Protein: 15g
- Fat: 10g

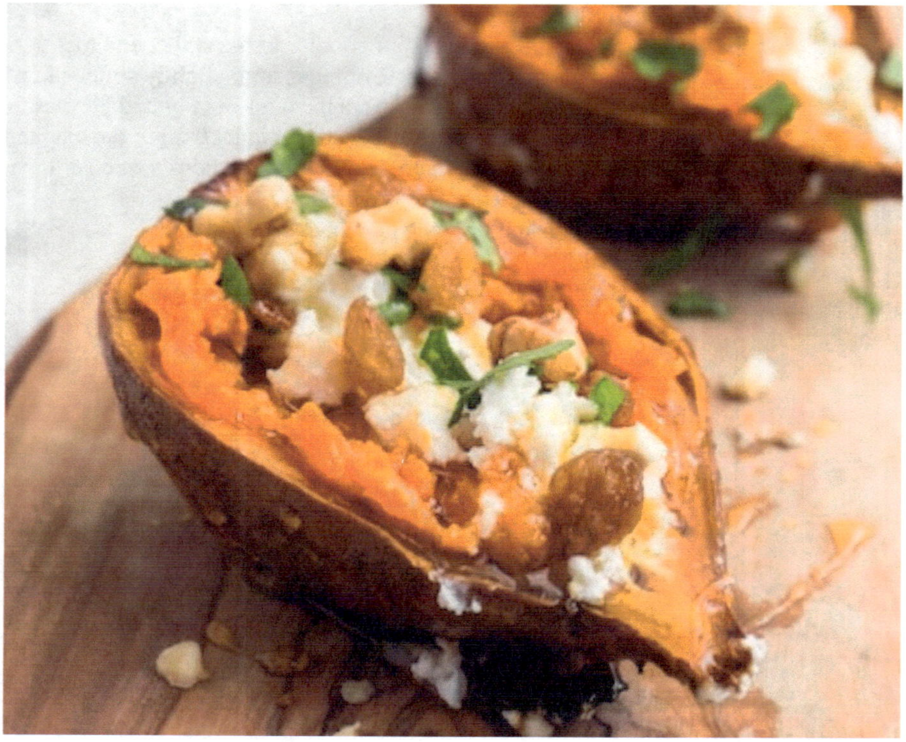

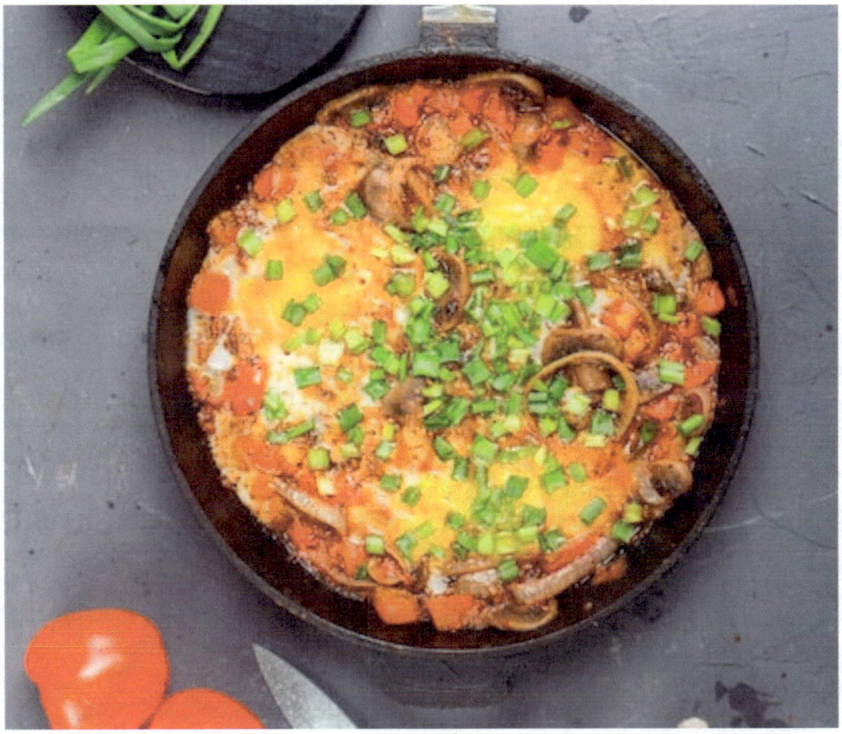

85. Eggplant and Chickpea Shakshuka

Prep.Time: 15 min

Cook Time: 25 min

Serving: 4

Beverage pairing: Lemonade

Ingredients:

- 1 large eggplant, diced
- 1 can (15 oz) chickpeas, drained and rinsed
- 1 onion, chopped
- 2 cloves garlic, minced
- 1 can (14 oz) diced tomatoes
- 1 teaspoon ground cumin
- 1 teaspoon smoked paprika
- 1/2 teaspoon ground coriander
- 1/4 teaspoon cayenne pepper (optional)
- Salt and pepper to taste
- 4 eggs
- Chopped fresh parsley for garnish

Preparation:

1. Heat olive oil in a large skillet over medium heat. Add chopped onion and diced eggplant. Cook until softened, about 5-7 minutes.
2. Add minced garlic to the skillet and cook for another minute until fragrant.
3. Stir in drained and rinsed chickpeas, diced tomatoes, ground cumin, smoked paprika, ground coriander, cayenne pepper (if using), salt, and pepper. Simmer for 10-15 minutes until the flavors meld together and the sauce thickens slightly.
4. Using a spoon, create wells in the sauce and crack one egg into each well.
5. Cover the skillet and cook for 5-7 minutes, or until the egg whites are set but the yolks are still runny.
6. Garnish with chopped fresh parsley before serving.
7. Serve hot with crusty bread or pita for dipping.

Nutrition Facts (per serving):

- Calories: 250
- Carbohydrates: 30g
- Protein: 12g
- Fat: 10g

86. Quinoa and Vegetable Stir-Fry with Cashews

Prep.Time: 15 min

Cook Time: 25 min

Serving: 4

Beverage pairing: Herbal Tea

Ingredients:

- 1 cup quinoa, rinsed
- 2 cups water or vegetable broth
- 2 tablespoons olive oil
- 2 cloves garlic, minced
- 1 onion, sliced
- 2 cups mixed vegetables (bell peppers, broccoli, carrots, snap peas, etc.), chopped
- 1/4 cup low-sodium soy sauce
- 2 tablespoons rice vinegar
- 1/2 cup unsalted cashews
- Salt and pepper to taste

Preparation:

1. In a saucepan, bring water or vegetable broth to a boil. Add quinoa, reduce heat to low, cover, and simmer for 15-20 minutes, or until quinoa is cooked and liquid is absorbed. Remove from heat and let it sit for 5 minutes, then fluff with a fork.
2. In a large skillet or wok, heat olive oil over medium-high heat. Add minced garlic and sliced onion, and cook until softened.
3. Add chopped mixed vegetables to the skillet and stir-fry for 5-6 minutes, or until vegetables are tender-crisp.
4. In a small bowl, whisk together low-sodium soy sauce, rice vinegar, and honey.
5. Pour the sauce over the vegetables in the skillet. Stir to coat evenly.
6. Add cooked quinoa and unsalted cashews to the skillet. Stir-fry for another 2-3 minutes to heat through.
7. Season with salt and pepper to taste.
8. Garnish with chopped green onions before serving.

Nutrition Facts (per serving):

- Calories: 300
- Carbs: 30g
- Protein: 10g
- Fat: 15g

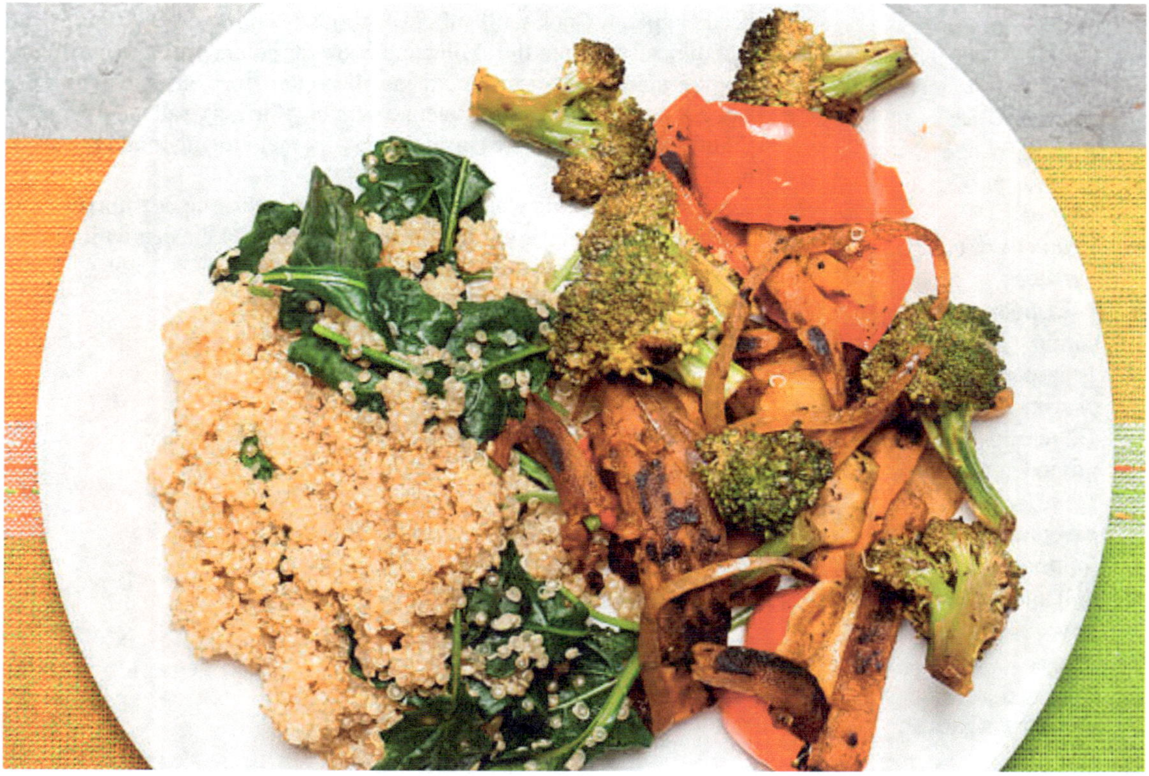

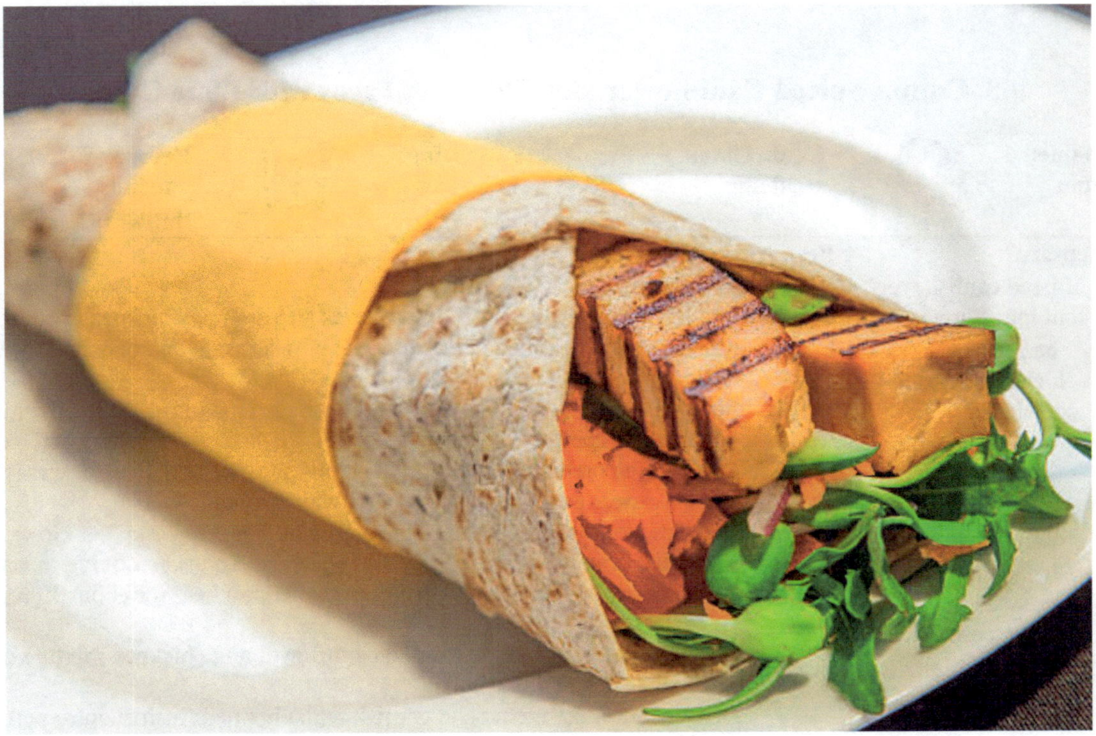

87. Grilled Tofu and Vegetable Wrap with Spicy Peanut Sauce

Prep.Time: 15 min

Cook Time: 10 min

Serving: 4

Beverage pairing: Herbal Tea

Ingredients:

- 1 block extra-firm tofu, sliced
- 4 whole wheat or low-carb wraps
- 2 cups mixed vegetables (bell peppers, zucchini, onions, mushrooms, etc.), sliced
- 2 tablespoons olive oil
- 1/4 cup natural peanut butter
- 2 tablespoons low-sodium soy sauce
- 1 tablespoon rice vinegar
- 1 tablespoon honey (or a sugar-free sweetener)
- 1 teaspoon sriracha sauce (adjust to taste)

Preparation:

1. Preheat grill to medium-high heat.
2. Brush sliced tofu and mixed vegetables with olive oil. Season with salt and pepper.
3. Grill tofu slices and mixed vegetables for 4-5 minutes per side, or until grill marks appear and they are heated through.
4. In a small bowl, whisk together natural peanut butter, low-sodium soy sauce, rice vinegar, honey, and sriracha sauce to make the spicy peanut sauce. Add water as needed to achieve desired consistency.
5. Lay out wraps and spread a generous amount of spicy peanut sauce on each wrap.
6. Arrange grilled tofu slices and mixed vegetables on top of the spicy peanut sauce on each wrap.
7. Roll up the wraps and cut in half if desired.
8. Garnish with chopped fresh cilantro before serving.

Nutrition Facts (per serving):

- Calories: 350
- Carbs: 30g
- Protein: 15g
- Fat: 20g

88. Cumin-Spiced Cauliflower and Chickpea Tacos with Lime Crema

Prep.Time: 15 min

Cook Time: 30 min

Serving: 4

Beverage pairing: Herbal Tea

Ingredients:

- 1 head cauliflower, cut into florets
- 1 can (15 oz) chickpeas, drained and rinsed
- 2 tablespoons olive oil
- 2 teaspoons ground cumin
- 1 teaspoon smoked paprika
- 1/2 teaspoon garlic powder
- Salt and pepper to taste
- 8 small corn tortillas
- 1/2 cup Greek yogurt
- Zest and juice of 1 lime

Preparation:

1. Preheat oven to 400°F (200°C).
2. In a large bowl, toss cauliflower florets and drained chickpeas with olive oil, ground cumin, smoked paprika, garlic powder, salt, and pepper until evenly coated.
3. Spread cauliflower and chickpea mixture on a baking sheet lined with parchment paper.
4. Roast in the preheated oven for 25-30 minutes, or until cauliflower is tender and chickpeas are crispy, stirring halfway through.
5. In the meantime, prepare the lime crema by whisking together Greek yogurt, lime zest, lime juice, and salt in a small bowl. Adjust seasoning to taste.
6. Warm corn tortillas in a dry skillet over medium heat for about 30 seconds on each side.
7. To assemble tacos, spoon roasted cauliflower and chickpea mixture onto warmed corn tortillas.
8. Drizzle with lime crema and garnish with chopped fresh cilantro before serving.

Nutrition Facts (per serving, serving size: 2 tacos):

- Calories: 300
- Carbs: 35g
- Protein: 10g
- Fat: 15g

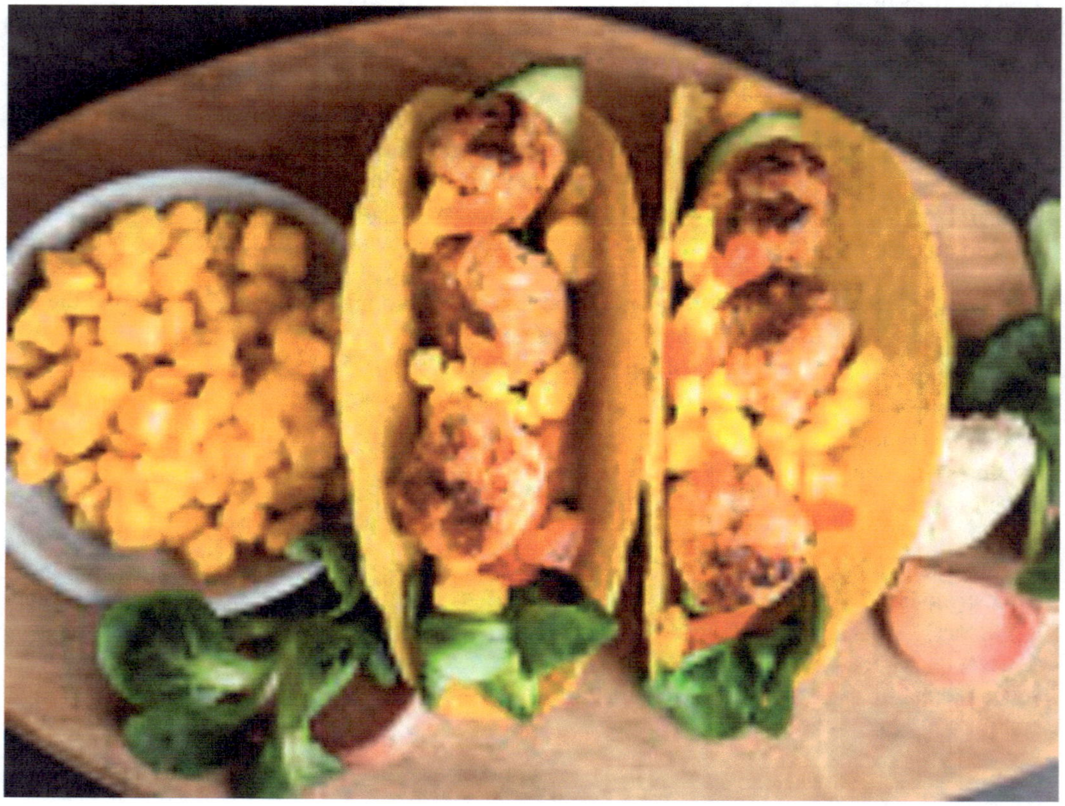

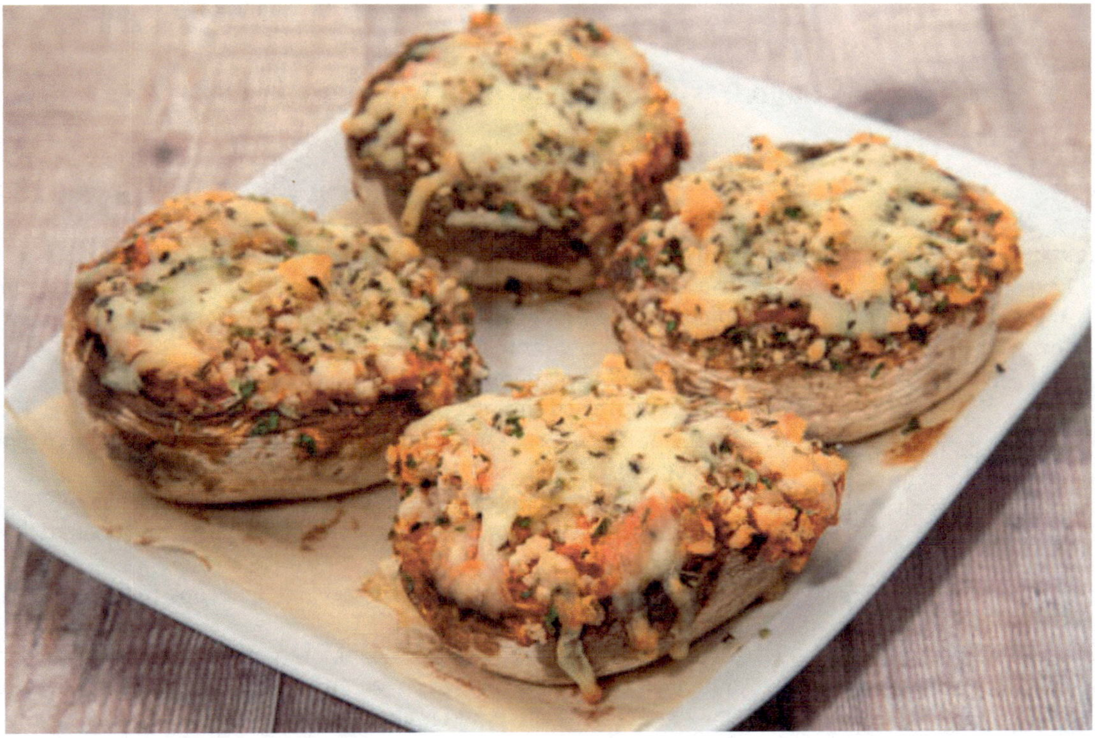

89. Turkey and Kale Stuffed Portobello Mushrooms

Prep.Time: 15 min

Cook Time: 25 min

Serving: 4

Beverage pairing: Herbal Tea

Ingredients:

- 4 large Portobello mushrooms, stems removed
- 1 pound ground turkey
- 2 cups chopped kale
- 1/2 cup diced onion
- 2 cloves garlic, minced
- 1 teaspoon dried thyme
- 1 teaspoon dried rosemary
- Salt and pepper to taste
- 1/4 cup grated Parmesan cheese (optional)
- Olive oil for brushing

Preparation:

1. Preheat oven to 375°F (190°C).
2. Brush Portobello mushrooms with olive oil and place them on a baking sheet lined with parchment paper.
3. In a skillet, cook ground turkey over medium heat until browned. Add diced onion and minced garlic, and cook until softened.
4. Stir in chopped kale, dried thyme, dried rosemary, salt, and pepper. Cook until kale is wilted.
5. Spoon the turkey and kale mixture into each Portobello mushroom cap.
6. Sprinkle grated Parmesan cheese on top of each stuffed mushroom if desired.
7. Bake in the preheated oven for 20-25 minutes, or until mushrooms are tender.
8. Serve hot.

Nutrition Facts (per serving):

- Calories: 250
- Carbs: 10g
- Protein: 25g
- Fat: 15g

90. Lemon Garlic Grilled Shrimp with Quinoa Pilaf

Prep.Time: 15 min

Cook Time: 20 min

Serving: 4

Beverage pairing: Iced Tea

Ingredients:

- 1 pound large shrimp, peeled and deveined
- Zest and juice of 1 lemon
- 2 cloves garlic, minced
- 2 tablespoons olive oil
- 1 cup quinoa, rinsed
- 2 cups low-sodium chicken broth
- 1 tablespoon olive oil
- 1 small onion, finely chopped
- 2 cloves garlic, minced
- 1/2 cup diced bell pepper
- 1/2 cup diced zucchini
- 1/4 cup chopped fresh parsley

Preparation:

1. In a bowl, combine peeled and deveined shrimp with lemon zest, lemon juice, minced garlic, olive oil, salt, and pepper. Toss until shrimp are evenly coated. Marinate for at least 15 minutes.
2. Preheat grill to medium-high heat.
3. Thread marinated shrimp onto skewers.
4. Grill shrimp skewers for 2-3 minutes per side, or until shrimp are pink and opaque.
5. In the meantime, prepare the quinoa pilaf. In a saucepan, heat olive oil over medium heat. Add chopped onion and minced garlic, and cook until softened.
6. Stir in diced bell pepper and diced zucchini, and cook for another 2-3 minutes.
7. Add rinsed quinoa and low-sodium chicken broth to the saucepan. Bring to a boil, then reduce heat to low, cover, and simmer for 15-20 minutes, or until quinoa is cooked and liquid is absorbed.
8. Remove quinoa pilaf from heat and stir in chopped fresh parsley. Season with salt and pepper to taste.
9. Serve grilled shrimp skewers with quinoa pilaf.

Nutrition Facts (per serving):

- Calories: 300
- Carbs: 30g
- Protein: 25g
- Fat: 10g

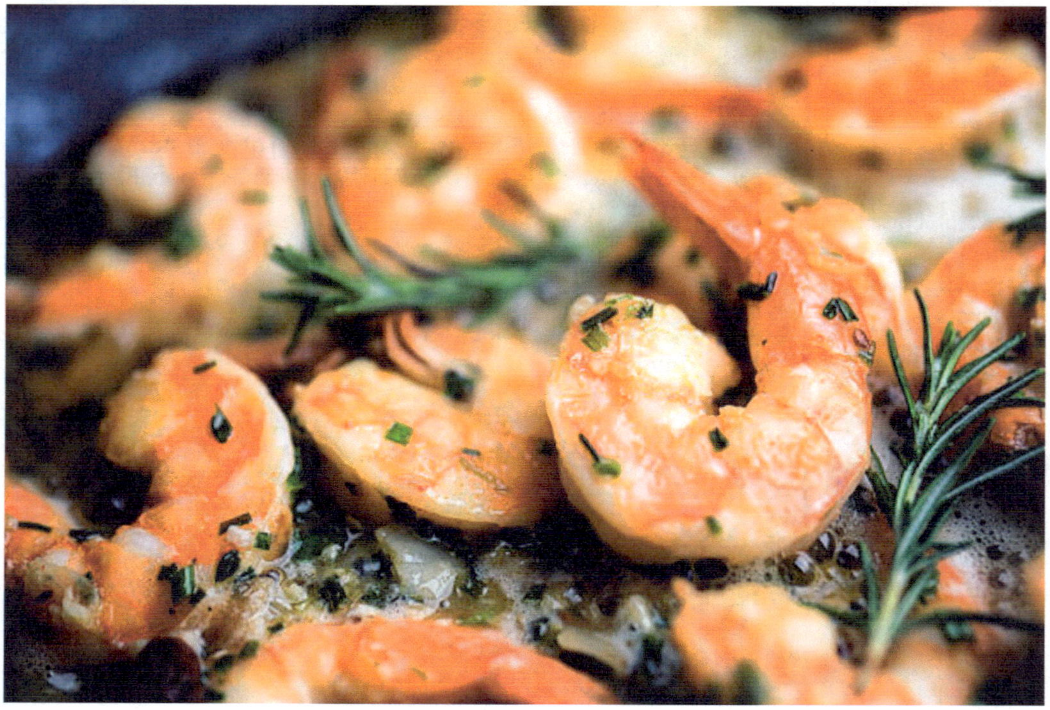

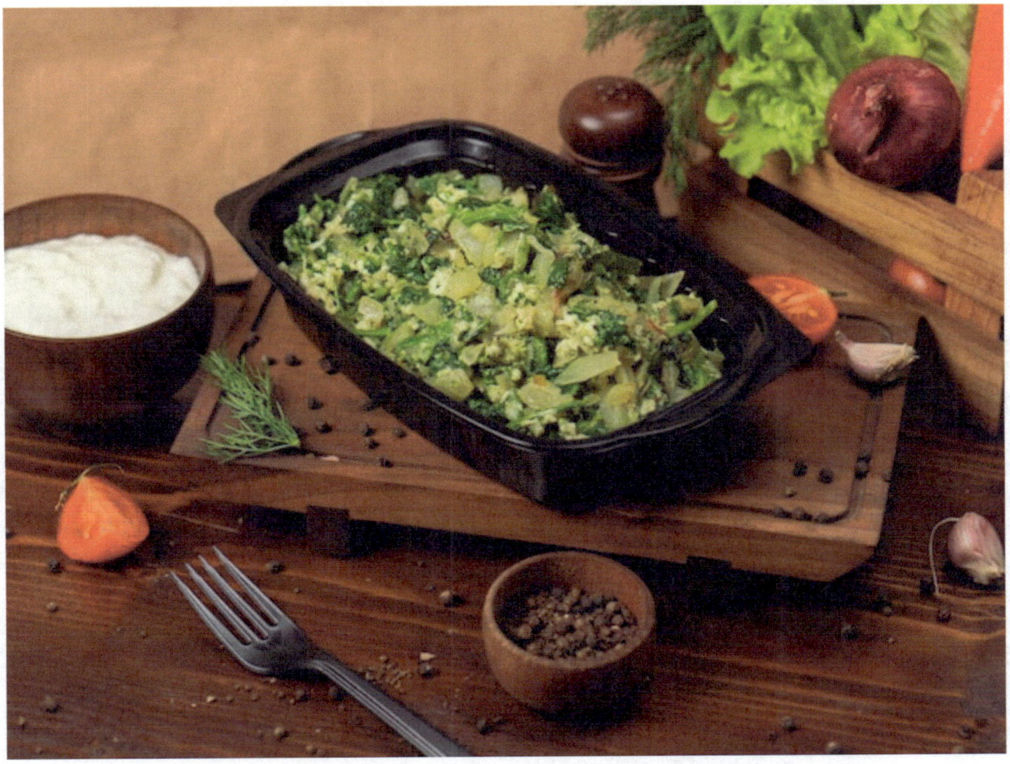

91. Cauliflower and Broccoli Mash with Parmesan

Prep.Time: 15 min

Cook Time: 10 min

Serving: 4

Beverage pairing: Herbal Tea

Ingredients:

- 1 head cauliflower, cut into florets
- 1 head broccoli, cut into florets
- 2 cloves garlic, minced
- 2 tablespoons olive oil
- 1/4 cup grated Parmesan cheese
- Salt and pepper to taste
- Chopped fresh parsley for garnish (optional)

Preparation:

1. Steam cauliflower and broccoli florets until tender.
2. In a skillet, heat olive oil over medium heat. Add minced garlic and cook until fragrant.
3. Add steamed cauliflower and broccoli to the skillet. Mash with a potato masher or fork until desired consistency is reached.
4. Stir in grated Parmesan cheese until melted and well combined.
5. Season with salt and pepper to taste.
6. Garnish with chopped fresh parsley before serving.

Nutrition Facts (per serving):

- Calories: 150
- Carbs: 10g
- Protein: 6g
- Fat: 10g

92. Spinach and Feta Stuffed Chicken Breast with Tomato Relish

Prep.Time: 15 min

Cook Time: 30 min

Serving: 4

Beverage pairing: Iced Tea

Ingredients:

- 4 boneless, skinless chicken breasts
- 2 cups fresh spinach leaves
- 1/2 cup crumbled feta cheese
- 1/4 cup chopped sun-dried tomatoes (packed in oil), drained
- 2 cloves garlic, minced
- Salt and pepper to taste
- Olive oil for brushing
- 1 cup cherry tomatoes, halved
- 1 tablespoon balsamic vinegar
- 1 tablespoon olive oil
- 1 tablespoon chopped fresh basil

Preparation:

1. Preheat oven to 375°F (190°C).
2. Place chicken breasts on a cutting board and make a horizontal slit along the side to create a pocket without cutting all the way through.
3. In a bowl, combine fresh spinach leaves, crumbled feta cheese, chopped sun-dried tomatoes, minced garlic, salt, and pepper.
4. Stuff each chicken breast with the spinach and feta mixture.
5. Brush stuffed chicken breasts with olive oil and season with additional salt and pepper if desired.
6. Place stuffed chicken breasts in a baking dish lined with parchment paper.
7. Bake in the preheated oven for 25-30 minutes, or until chicken is cooked through and juices run clear.
8. In the meantime, prepare the tomato relish by combining halved cherry tomatoes, balsamic vinegar, olive oil, chopped fresh basil, salt, and pepper in a bowl. Let it sit for flavors to meld.
9. Serve stuffed chicken breasts with tomato relish on top.

Nutrition Facts (per serving):

- Calories: 250
- Carbs: 5g
- Protein: 30g
- Fat: 10g

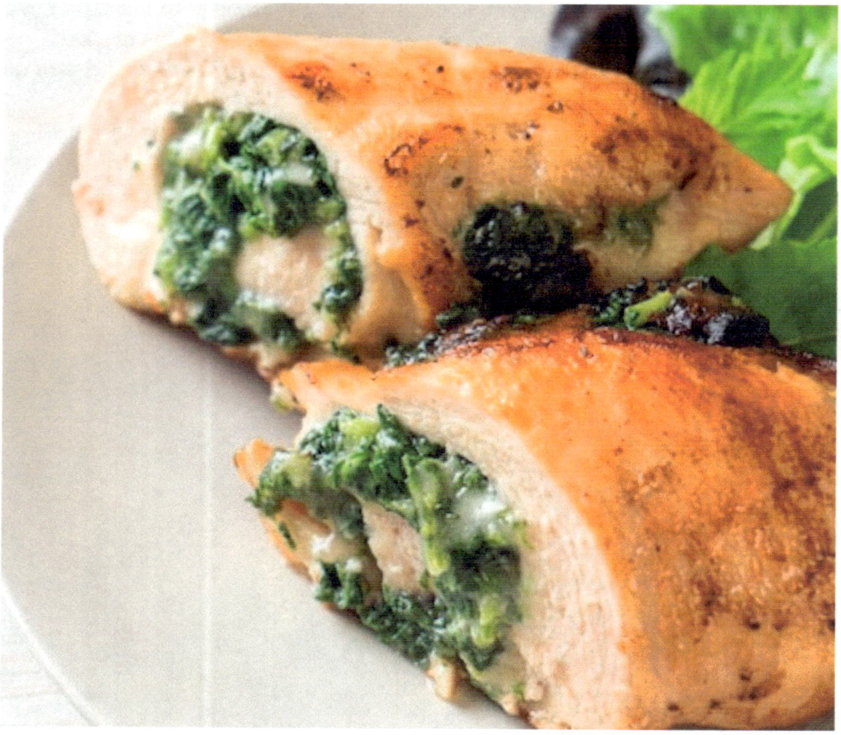

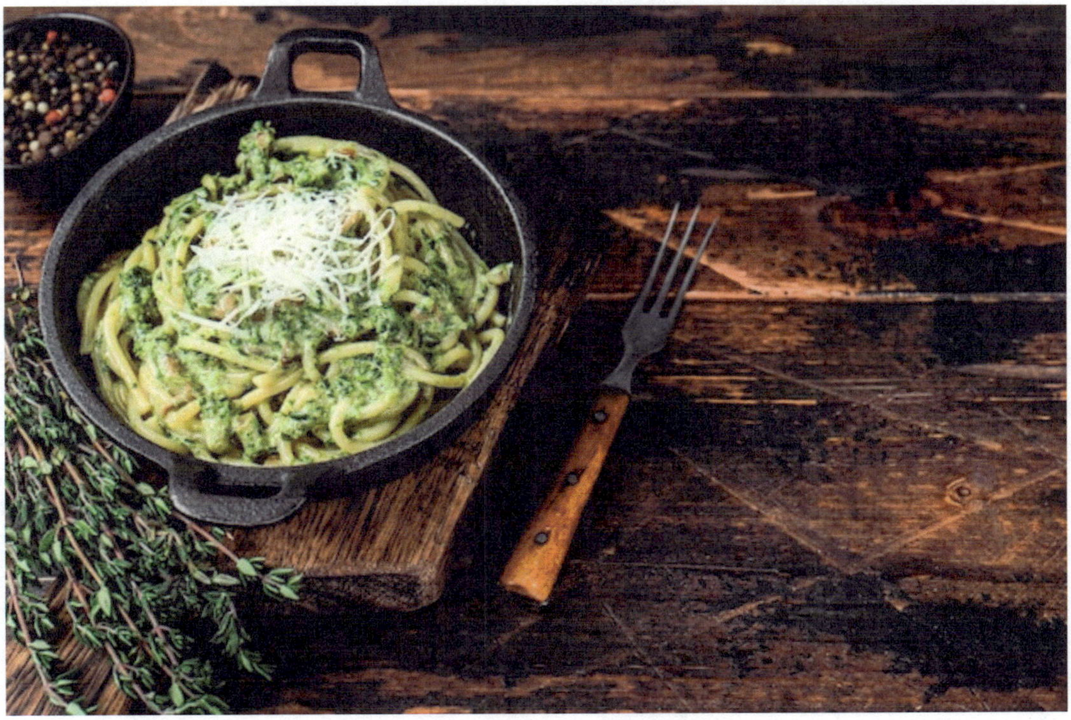

93. Mediterranean Zoodle (Zucchini Noodle) Bowl with Greek Yogurt Tzatziki

Prep.Time: 15 min

Cook Time: 0 min

Serving: 4

Beverage pairing: Herbal Tea

Ingredients:

- 4 medium zucchinis, spiralized into noodles
- 1 cup cherry tomatoes, halved
- 1/2 cup diced cucumber
- 1/4 cup sliced Kalamata olives
- 1/4 cup crumbled feta cheese
- 2 tablespoons chopped fresh parsley
- 1 cup Greek yogurt
- 1/2 cucumber, grated and squeezed to remove excess moisture
- 2 cloves garlic, minced
- 1 tablespoon chopped fresh dill

Preparation:

1. In a bowl, combine spiralized zucchini noodles, halved cherry tomatoes, diced cucumber, sliced Kalamata olives, crumbled feta cheese, and chopped fresh parsley.
2. In another bowl, prepare the Greek yogurt tzatziki by combining Greek yogurt, grated cucumber, minced garlic, lemon juice, chopped fresh dill, salt, and pepper. Mix until well combined.
3. Toss the zucchini noodle mixture with Greek yogurt tzatziki until evenly coated.
4. Divide the Mediterranean zoodle mixture into serving bowls.
5. Serve chilled or at room temperature.

Nutrition Facts (per serving):

- Calories: 150
- Carbs: 15g
- Protein: 10g
- Fat: 8g

94. Teriyaki Tofu and Broccoli Quinoa Bowl

Prep.Time: 15 min

Cook Time: 10 min

Serving: 4

Beverage pairing: Herbal Tea

Ingredients:

- 1 block extra-firm tofu, cubed
- 2 cups broccoli florets
- 1 cup cooked quinoa
- 2 tablespoons low-sodium soy sauce
- 2 tablespoons teriyaki sauce (look for a low-sugar option)
- 1 tablespoon rice vinegar
- 1 tablespoon sesame oil
- 2 cloves garlic, minced

Preparation:

1. In a bowl, combine cubed tofu, broccoli florets, cooked quinoa, low-sodium soy sauce, teriyaki sauce, rice vinegar, honey, sesame oil, and minced garlic. Toss until tofu and broccoli are evenly coated.
2. Heat a skillet over medium-high heat. Add tofu and broccoli mixture to the skillet.
3. Stir-fry for 5-6 minutes, or until tofu is browned and broccoli is tender-crisp.
4. Sprinkle sesame seeds and chopped green onions on top for garnish if desired.
5. Serve hot.

Nutrition Facts (per serving):

- Calories: 300
- Carbs: 35g
- Protein: 15g
- Fat: 12g

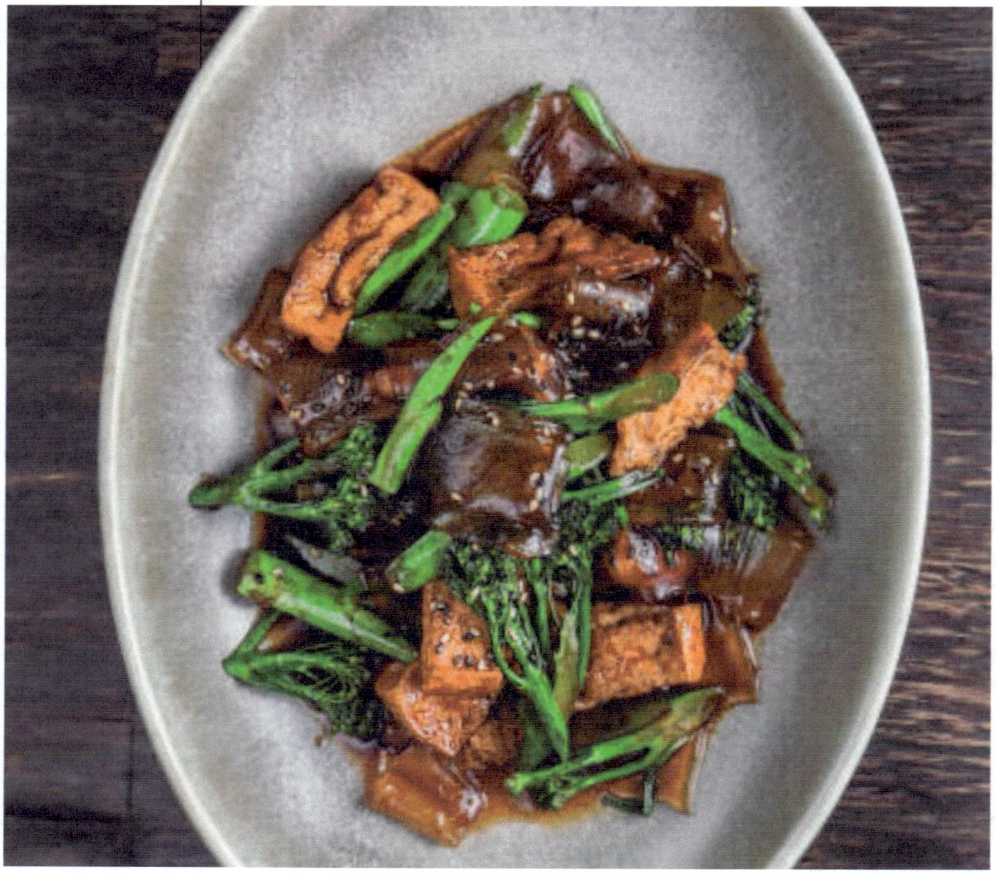

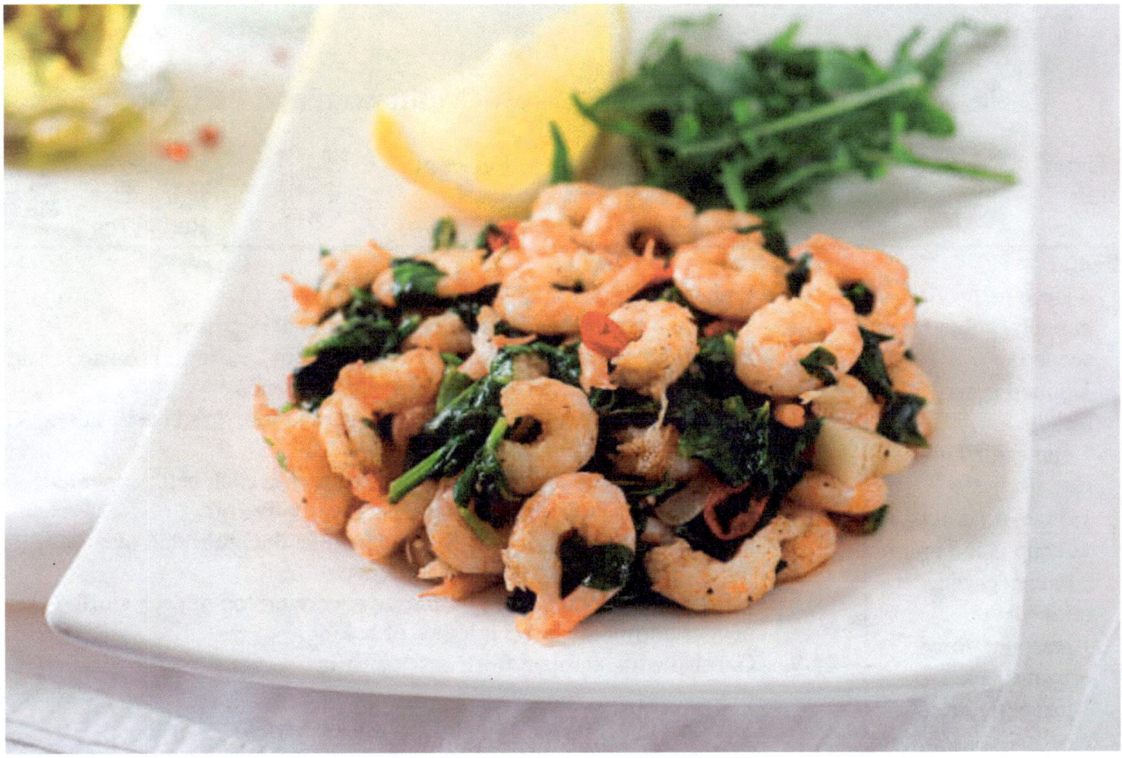

95. Lemon Garlic Shrimp with Spinach and Walnut Salad

Prep.Time: 15 min

Cook Time: 10 min

Serving: 4

Beverage pairing: Herbal Tea

Ingredients:

- 1 pound large shrimp, peeled and deveined
- Zest and juice of 1 lemon
- 2 cloves garlic, minced
- 2 tablespoons olive oil
- Salt and pepper to taste
- 4 cups fresh baby spinach leaves
- 1/2 cup chopped walnuts
- 2 tablespoons olive oil
- 1 tablespoon balsamic vinegar
- 1 teaspoon Dijon mustard

Preparation:

1. In a bowl, combine peeled and deveined shrimp with lemon zest, lemon juice, minced garlic, olive oil, salt, and pepper. Toss until shrimp are evenly coated. Marinate for at least 15 minutes.
2. Heat a skillet over medium-high heat. Add marinated shrimp to the skillet.
3. Cook shrimp for 2-3 minutes per side, or until pink and opaque.
4. In a large salad bowl, combine fresh baby spinach leaves and chopped walnuts.
5. In a small bowl, whisk together olive oil, balsamic vinegar, Dijon mustard, salt, and pepper to make the salad dressing.
6. Drizzle salad dressing over the spinach and walnut mixture. Toss until evenly coated.
7. Divide the spinach and walnut salad into serving plates.
8. Top each salad with lemon garlic shrimp.
9. Serve immediately.

Nutrition Facts (per serving):

- Calories: 250
- Carbs: 8g
- Protein: 25g
- Fat: 15g

96. Stuffed Bell Peppers with Turkey, Cauliflower, and Pine Nuts

Prep.Time: 15 min

Cook Time: 35 min

Serving: 4

Beverage pairing: Herbal Tea

Ingredients:

- 4 large bell peppers, halved and seeded
- 1 pound ground turkey
- 1 cup cauliflower rice
- 1/4 cup pine nuts
- 1/2 cup diced onion
- 2 cloves garlic, minced
- 1 teaspoon dried oregano
- 1 teaspoon dried basil
- Salt and pepper to taste
- Olive oil for brushing

Preparation:

1. Preheat oven to 375°F (190°C).
2. Place halved and seeded bell peppers in a baking dish.
3. In a skillet, cook ground turkey over medium heat until browned. Add diced onion and minced garlic, and cook until softened.
4. Stir in cauliflower rice, pine nuts, dried oregano, dried basil, salt, and pepper. Cook until cauliflower rice is tender.
5. Spoon the turkey and cauliflower mixture into each bell pepper half.
6. Brush the tops of stuffed bell peppers with olive oil.
7. Cover the baking dish with foil and bake in the preheated oven for 30-35 minutes, or until bell peppers are tender.
8. If desired, sprinkle grated Parmesan cheese on top of each stuffed bell pepper during the last 5 minutes of baking.
9. Garnish with chopped fresh parsley before serving.

Nutrition Facts (per serving):

- Calories: 300
- Carbs: 15g
- Protein: 25g
- Fat: 15g

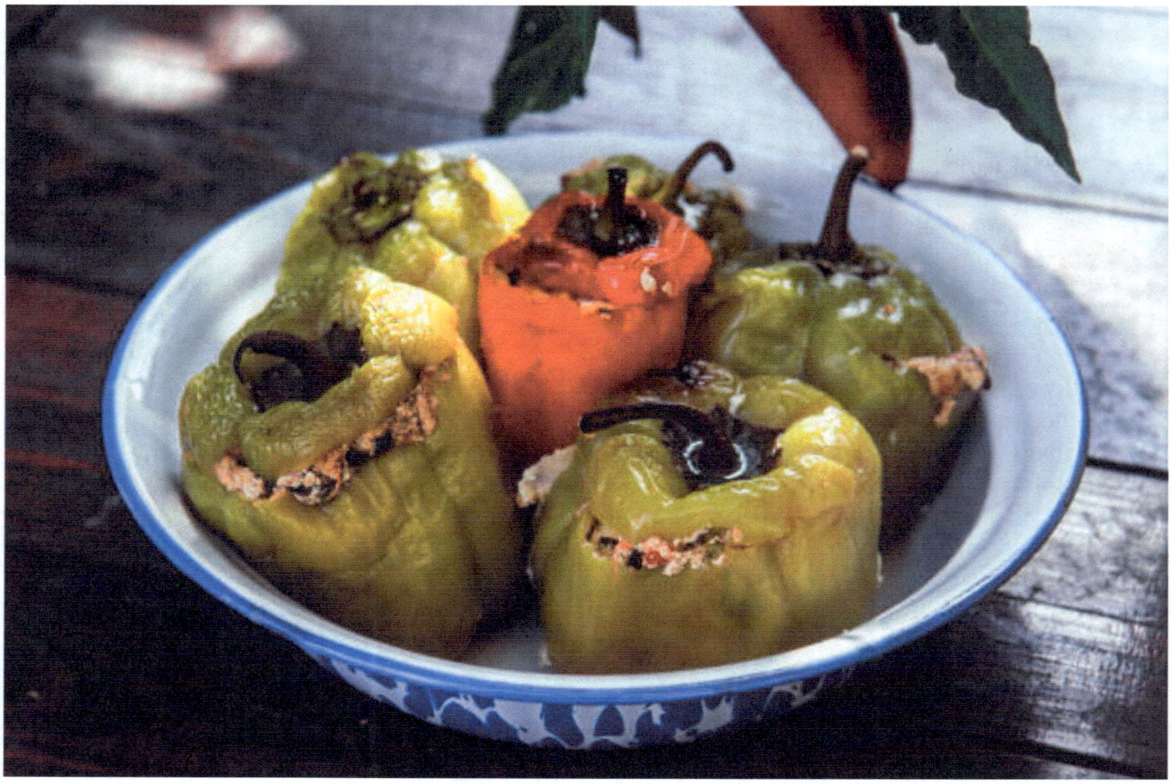

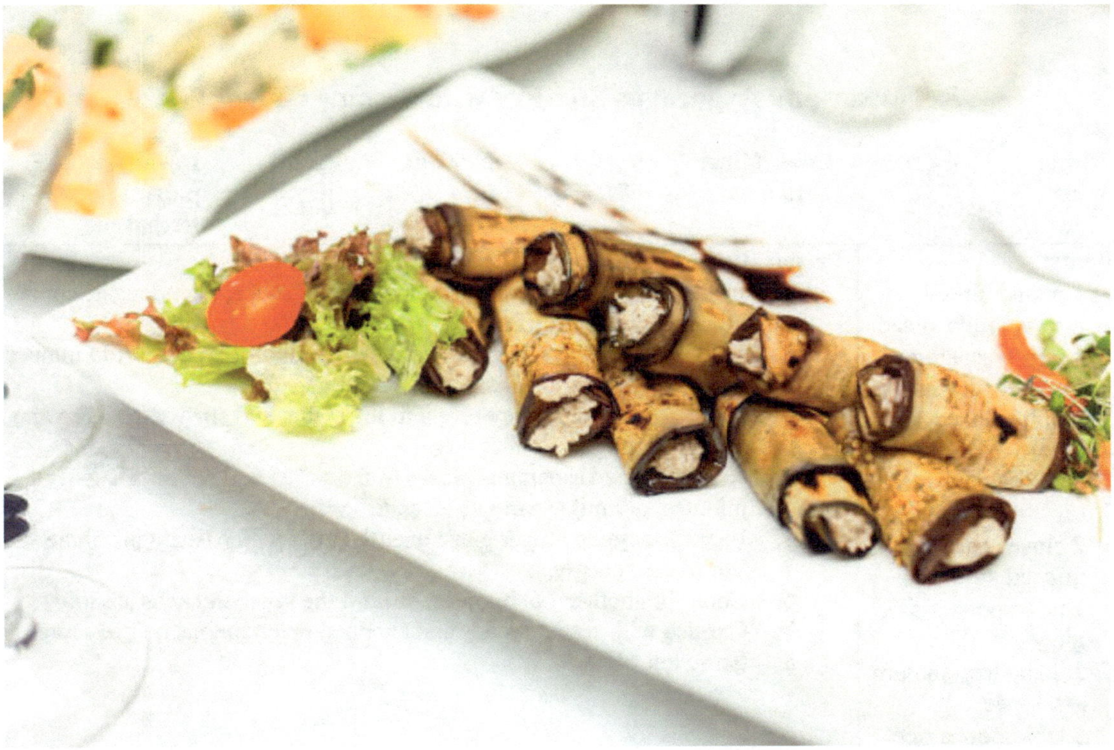

97. Grilled Eggplant and Zucchini Roll-Ups with Tomato Basil Sauce

Prep.Time: 15 min

Cook Time: 15 min

Serving: 4

Beverage pairing: Herbal Tea

Ingredients:

- 1 large eggplant, sliced lengthwise into thin strips
- 2 medium zucchinis, sliced lengthwise into thin strips
- 2 tablespoons olive oil
- Salt and pepper to taste
- 1 can (14 oz) crushed tomatoes
- 2 cloves garlic, minced
- 1 tablespoon olive oil
- 1 teaspoon dried basil

Preparation:

1. Preheat grill to medium-high heat.
2. Brush eggplant and zucchini strips with olive oil. Season with salt and pepper.
3. Grill eggplant and zucchini strips for 2-3 minutes per side, or until tender and grill marks appear.
4. In the meantime, prepare the tomato basil sauce. In a saucepan, heat olive oil over medium heat. Add minced garlic and cook until fragrant.
5. Stir in crushed tomatoes, dried basil, salt, and pepper. Simmer for 5-7 minutes, stirring occasionally.
6. Place a spoonful of tomato basil sauce on each grilled eggplant and zucchini strip.
7. Roll up the eggplant and zucchini strips and secure with toothpicks if needed.
8. Serve grilled eggplant and zucchini roll-ups with additional tomato basil sauce on the side.

Nutrition Facts (per serving):

- Calories: 150
- Carbs: 10g
- Protein: 3g
- Fat: 10g

98. Turkey and Asparagus Stir-Fry with Sesame Ginger Glaze

Prep.Time: 15 min

Cook Time: 15 min

Serving: 4

Beverage pairing: Herbal Tea

Ingredients:

- 1 pound turkey breast, thinly sliced
- 1 bunch asparagus, trimmed and cut into bite-sized pieces
- 2 tablespoons olive oil
- 2 cloves garlic, minced
- 1 tablespoon grated ginger
- 1/4 cup low-sodium soy sauce
- 2 tablespoons rice vinegar
- 1 tablespoon honey (or a sugar-free sweetener)
- 1 teaspoon sesame oil

Preparation:

1. In a bowl, whisk together low-sodium soy sauce, rice vinegar, honey, sesame oil, and cornstarch (if using). Set aside.
2. Heat olive oil in a skillet or wok over medium-high heat. Add minced garlic and grated ginger, and cook until fragrant.
3. Add thinly sliced turkey breast to the skillet and stir-fry until browned and cooked through.
4. Add bite-sized asparagus pieces to the skillet and continue stir-frying for 3-4 minutes, or until asparagus is tender-crisp.
5. Pour the sesame ginger glaze over the turkey and asparagus in the skillet. Stir to coat evenly.
6. Cook for another 1-2 minutes, or until the sauce thickens slightly.
7. Garnish with sesame seeds and chopped green onions before serving.
8. Serve hot.

Nutrition Facts (per serving):

- Calories: 250
- Carbs: 10g
- Protein: 30g
- Fat: 10g

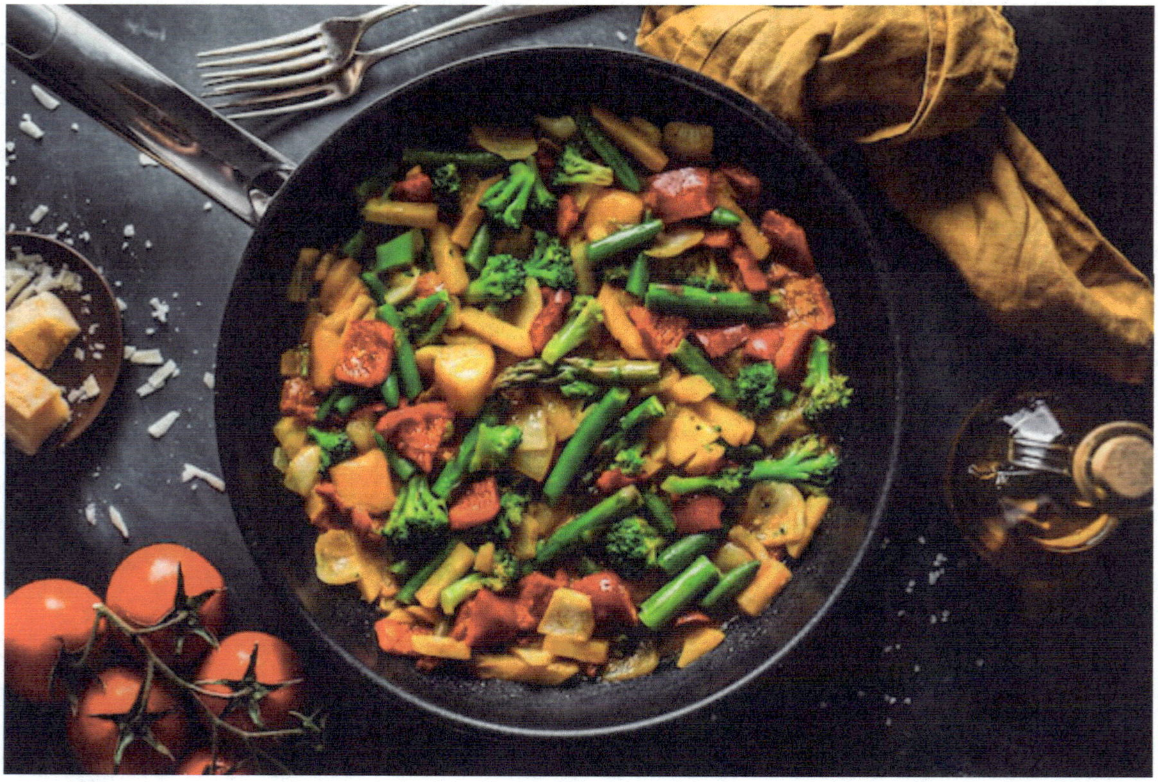

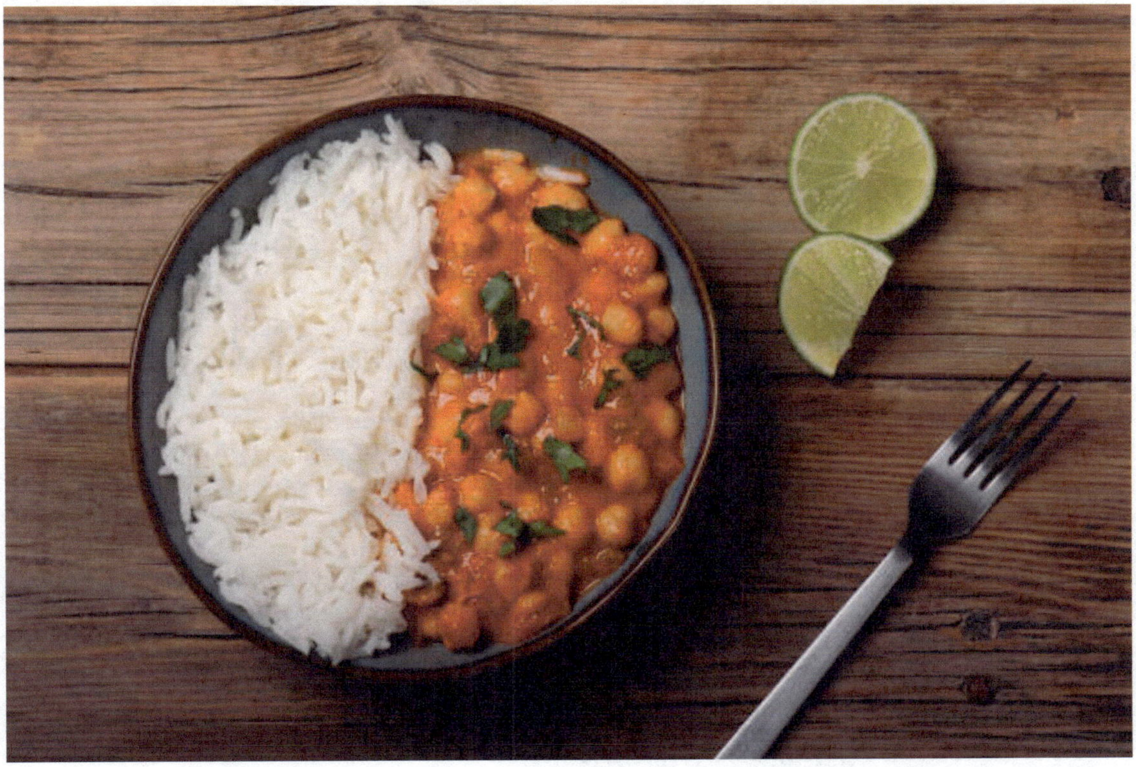

99. Chickpea and Vegetable Curry with Cilantro Lime Cauliflower Rice

Prep.Time: 15 min

Cook Time: 20 min

Serving: 4

Beverage pairing: Herbal Tea

Ingredients:

- 1 can (15 oz) chickpeas, drained and rinsed
- 2 cups mixed vegetables (bell peppers, carrots, peas, etc.), chopped
- 1 onion, diced
- 2 cloves garlic, minced
- 1 tablespoon grated ginger
- 1 can (14 oz) coconut milk
- 2 tablespoons curry powder
- 1/2 teaspoon ground cumin
- Chopped fresh cilantro for garnish
- 1 head cauliflower, grated
- 1/4 cup chopped fresh cilantro

Preparation:

1. In a large skillet or pot, heat olive oil over medium heat. Add diced onion, minced garlic, and grated ginger, and cook until softened.
2. Add chopped mixed vegetables to the skillet and cook for 5-6 minutes, or until vegetables are tender.
3. Stir in drained and rinsed chickpeas, curry powder, ground turmeric, ground cumin, salt, and pepper.
4. Pour coconut milk into the skillet and stir to combine. Bring to a simmer and cook for 10-12 minutes, stirring occasionally.
5. In the meantime, prepare the cilantro lime cauliflower rice. In a separate skillet, heat olive oil over medium heat. Add grated cauliflower and cook for 5-6 minutes, or until cauliflower is tender.
6. Remove from heat and stir in lime zest, lime juice, chopped fresh cilantro, and salt.
7. Serve chickpea and vegetable curry over cilantro lime cauliflower rice.
8. Garnish with chopped fresh cilantro before serving.

Nutrition Facts (per serving):

- Calories: 300
- Carbs: 25g
- Protein: 10g
- Fat: 15g

100. Baked Salmon with Dill and Roasted Brussels Sprouts

Prep.Time: 15 min

Cook Time: 20 min

Serving: 4

Beverage pairing: Herbal Tea

Ingredients:

- 4 salmon fillets
- 2 tablespoons olive oil
- 2 tablespoons chopped fresh dill
- Zest and juice of 1 lemon
- 2 cloves garlic, minced
- Salt and pepper to taste
- 1 pound Brussels sprouts, trimmed and halved
- 1 tablespoon balsamic vinegar

Preparation:

1. Preheat oven to 400°F (200°C).
2. Place salmon fillets on a baking sheet lined with parchment paper.
3. In a bowl, whisk together olive oil, chopped fresh dill, lemon zest, lemon juice, minced garlic, salt, and pepper.
4. Brush the dill mixture over the salmon fillets.
5. In another bowl, toss halved Brussels sprouts with olive oil, balsamic vinegar, honey, salt, and pepper until evenly coated.
6. Spread Brussels sprouts in a single layer on the baking sheet around the salmon fillets.
7. Bake in the preheated oven for 15-20 minutes, or until salmon is cooked through and Brussels sprouts are tender.
8. Serve hot.

Nutrition Facts (per serving):

- Calories: 300
- Carbs: 15g
- Protein: 30g
- Fat: 15g

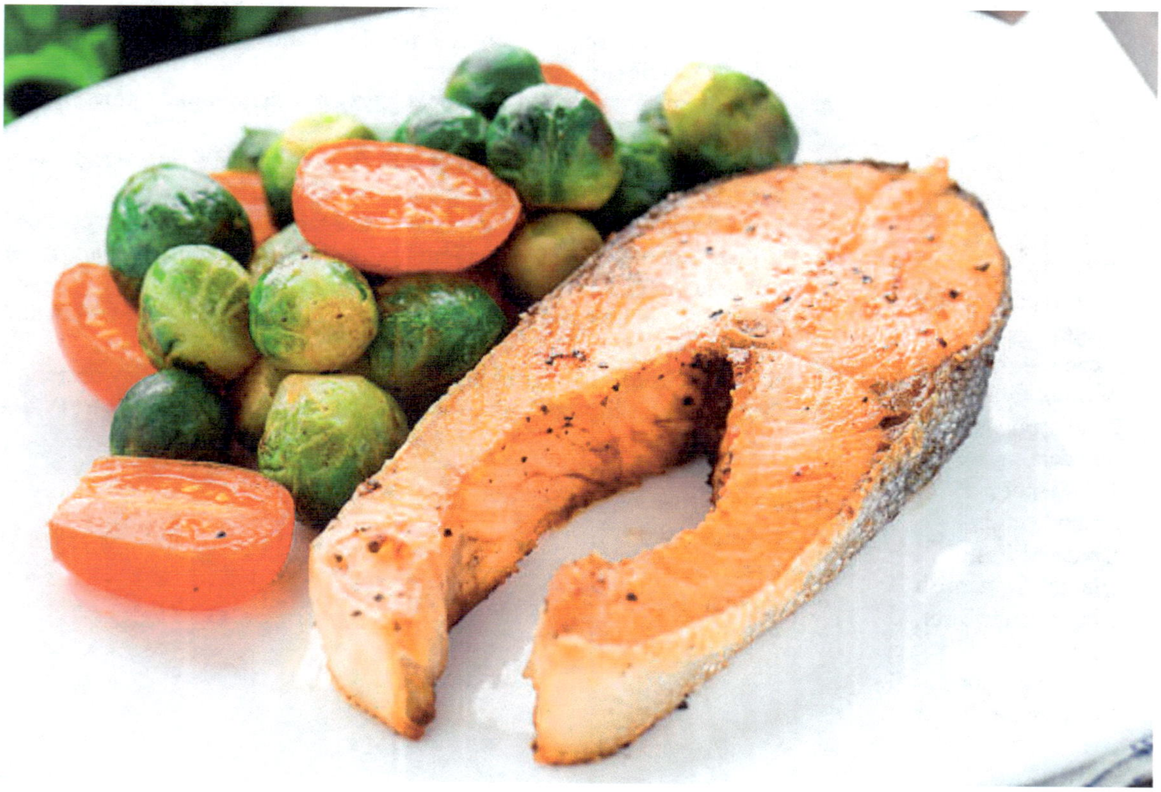

Sharing Your Culinary Journey

Now that you've mastered the art of creating delicious, diabetes-friendly meals, it's time to share your newfound culinary wisdom with others who are on the same path. By leaving your honest review of the "Type 2 Diabetes Cookbook: Beginner's Quick & Easy Recipes for Delicious Diabetes Diets" by Lily Anders on Amazon, you'll guide fellow food enthusiasts to a resource that can transform their dining table and health.

Your insights and experiences are invaluable, offering a beacon to those navigating their diet amidst diabetes. Whether it was a specific recipe that became your go-to, a tip that changed how you approach cooking, or the overall ease and enjoyment you found in these pages, your feedback is a gift that keeps on giving.

Thank you for contributing to a community of knowledge and support. The journey towards healthy eating and diabetes management thrives on shared discoveries and successes. By passing on your review, you're not just recommending a book—you're enriching lives with the joy of cooking and the empowerment of dietary control.

To leave your review, just follow this link:

https://www.amazon.com/review/create-review/?ie=UTF8&channel=glance-detail&asin=1963939336

Together, we're keeping the passion for healthy, joyful eating alive, one review at a time. Your support makes all the difference, not just to us, but to every reader and cook who seeks to balance their love for food with their health needs.

- With heartfelt thanks,

Lily Anders

Conclusion

In conclusion, this book transcends the traditional approach to managing diabetes through diet alone, offering a comprehensive guide that empowers individuals with diabetes to navigate their condition with knowledge and precision. Through 300 carefully crafted recipes, we explore the importance of balancing nutrient intake and the vital role of consistent meal planning. Each recipe is not just a set of instructions but a building block towards a healthier life, tailored to the unique needs of those managing diabetes.

As we close this journey of understanding and adaptation, remember that managing diabetes is not just about adhering to dietary restrictions or grappling with numbers—it is about reclaiming control of your health and life. These recipes are designed not only to meet specific nutritional needs but also to delight the palate, proving that a diabetes-conscious diet can be as delicious as it is nutritious.

Embrace these culinary tools as your allies in the pursuit of wellness. Let each meal enrich your body and spirit, and may the knowledge contained in this book guide you toward a balanced, joyful, and healthy life with diabetes. Here's to finding pleasure in every bite and strength in every challenge. Cheers to your health and happiness on this flavorful journey!

Made in United States
Cleveland, OH
05 November 2026

47768322R00073